CALVERT'S DESCRIPTIVE PHONETICS TRANSCRIPTION WORKBOOK

Third Edition

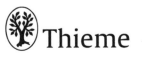

CALVERT'S DESCRIPTIVE PHONETICS TRANSCRIPTION WORKBOOK

Third Edition

Pamela Garn-Nunn, Ph.D.
Professor
School of Speech-Language Pathology and Audiology
University of Akron
Akron, OH

James M. Lynn, Ph.D.
Associate Dean
College of Fine and Applied Arts
University of Akron
Akron, OH

Thieme

New York • Stuttgart

Thieme Medical Publishers, Inc.
333 Seventh Ave.
New York, NY 10001

Director, Production and Manufacturing: Anne Vinnicombe
Production Editor: Becky Dille
Marketing Director: Phyllis Gold
Sales Manager: Ross Lumpkin
Chief Financial Officer: Peter van Woerden
President: Brian D. Scanlan
Compositor: Compset, Inc.
Printer: Maple-Vail Book Manufacturing Group
Library of Congress Cataloging-in-Publication Data

Important note: Medical knowledge is ever-changing. As new research and clinical experience broaden our knowledge, changes in treatment and drug therapy may be required. The authors and editors of the material herein have consulted sources believed to be reliable in their efforts to provide information that is complete and in accord with the standards accepted at the time of publication. However, in the view of the possibility of human error by the authors, editors, or publisher, of the work herein, or changes in medical knowledge, neither the authors, editors, or publisher, nor any other party who has been involved in the preparation of this work, warrants that the information contained herein is in every respect accurate or complete, and they are not responsible for any errors or omissions or for the results obtained from use of such information. Readers are encouraged to confirm the information contained herein with other sources. For example, readers are advised to check the product information sheet included in the package of each drug they plan to administer to be certain that the information contained in this publication is accurate and that changes have not been made in the recommended dose or in the contraindications for administration. This recommendation is of particular importance in connection with new or infrequently used drugs.

Some of the product names, patents, and registered designs referred to in this book are in fact registered trademarks or proprietary names even though specific reference to this fact is not always made in the text. Therefore, the appearance of a name without designation as proprietary is not to be construed as a representation by the publisher that it is in the public domain.

Printed in the United States of America
5 4 3 2 1
TMP ISBN 1-58890-018-5
GTV ISBN 3 13 617203 5

CONTENTS

PART 5   MARKINGS FOR SPEECH RHYTHM

PART 6   DIALECTIC VARIATIONS

FOREWORD TO THE INSTRUCTOR

This transcription workbook, like previous editions, has been designed for use in conjunction with *Calvert's Descriptive Phonetics,* third edition. It may also be used alone or in conjunction with a different textbook. Most importantly, it should be used as one component of an academic course that includes lecture, examples, and many opportunities for transcription practice. Instructors may wish to use all, or only parts, of this workbook. Coverage should require approximately a year of course work, depending on the pace of instruction and the number of content areas included in the course.

ADDITIONS TO THE WORKBOOK

We have added a chapter to help you prepare students to think in terms of phonemes rather than alphabetic letters. In our experience, students frequently tend to think or see words in terms of letters, e.g., *back* as four letters, rather than in terms of phonemes, /bæk/ as three phonemes. Their confusion should not be surprising when we consider that previous years of schooling emphasized reading and writing with the alphabet. Some students find it more difficult than others to make the transition back to thinking in terms of auditory images rather than alphabetic representations. Consequently, Chapter 1 in this edition of the workbook has been added to help students reorient their thinking. We have also included additional transcription exercises in the chapters on vowels and diphthongs. [An instructional CD can also be used in conjunction with Parts 1, 2, and 3.]

ORGANIZATIONAL CHANGES

In Chapters 2 through 10 (Vowels, Diphthongs, Consonants), we have maintained sections from previous editions to help students develop skills in phoneme recognition, discrimination, and word transcription. In Recognition, the student must identify the phoneme common to a given list of words. Discrimination exercises require the student to determine which words contain a given target phoneme. [These exercises can be completed with the instructional CD or through in-class exercises presented by the instructor.]

Chapters 2 through 10 also include exercises that require a higher level of listening skill and actual International Phonetic Alphabet (IPA) transcription. Section C, Word Transcription from Spelling/Dictation, is intended for further practice prior to completing the final, live transcription exercise (Exercise D) in each chapter. We do not recommend that the student read and pronounce aloud words in order to transcribe these exercises. Pronunciation of some vowels can vary widely according to a student's regional dialect and/or ethnic background. Consequently, we recommend that exercises be presented aloud by an instructor (lists provided).

This should allow students to build a consistent auditory image and transcription competence before dealing with pronunciation variations (see Chapters 6 and 8 in the text and Part 6 in this workbook). Of course, the final choice for using these exercises is the instructor's.

We also changed the sequencing of consonant and vowel presentation. Vowels are now covered before consonants in both text and workbook. Again, in our experience, students have more difficulty learning the vowels (i.e., their "alphabet letter orientation") than the consonants. Putting vowels first allows additional vowel practice not afforded in previous editions. Actual students' feedback (to the second author, who regularly teaches an undergraduate phonetics course) has repeatedly supported learning vowels first. If you have a different preference, feel free to choose your own order of presentation.

As in previous editions, the third primary area of focus in this workbook is narrow transcription. We have made some changes in the grouping of these chapters, but their content remains the same.

Overall, our goal in revising this workbook was to provide students with multiple opportunities to learn IPA symbols and apply them in transcription. Repeated listening and transcription practice are the keys to proficiency with the IPA. Such exercises are only a tool, however; they require a skilled instructor to make them useful and to facilitate actual student learning. We hope that you find this new edition as useful as previous editions.

We wish to thank Phil Hoffman for his able assistance in developing the compact disk. He recorded all the word lists, and also served as technical consultant. Mr. Hoffman is manager of the media production facilities, School of Communication at The University of Akron.

P G G-N
J M L

PART 1

INTRODUCTION

BACKGROUND: PHONETIC TRANSCRIPTION

Phonetic transcription is a part of the study of descriptive phonetics that relates both to linguistics and to speech science. As you might imagine, it is an essential skill for scholars in either of these disciplines. It also has numerous practical applications for individuals interested in a variety of areas, such as

- Speech communication through a variety of electronic media
- Dramatic arts
- Speech-language pathology and audiology
- Teaching speech to children who are deaf or have a language disorder
- Teaching English as a second language (ESL)
- Teaching foreign languages to native English speakers
- Teaching children who are bilingual
- Teaching reading by a phonics approach

Development of actual accurate phonetic transcription skills requires care, practice, and relearning to listen. As a child developing language, you learned to focus more on message content than on possible variations in pronunciation or speech sounds. You developed the ability to understand words and sentences regardless of speaker (e.g., child or adult), phonetic context, and individual variations in pronunciation.

Most likely, you will need to inhibit some of these influences on the way you "hear" sounds in order to develop accurate transcription skills. For example, dialectic variations are found in speakers of different regions and ethnic groups. If your dialect varies from the mainstream (general) American English that is the reference for this workbook and companion textbook, you will have to reorient your listening. For example, pronunciation of the vowel in *aunt* can vary according to your dialect. You may pronounce it as *ahnt* (East Coast), *ant* (Midwest), or *aint* (South, Appalachia). Each of these pronunciations is correct for the region in which it is used. But if you're used to saying and hearing *aunt* as *ahnt*, you may have difficulty hearing your instructor's mainstream American English pronunciation of the word as *ant*. This workbook is designed to give you many opportunities to practice listening for such variations in pronunciation.

Another influence on your ability to develop accurate phonetic transcription skills comes from learning to read and write. We tend to "see" words in terms of spelling and its determination of pronunciation. In reality, spelling and pronunciation often are only poorly related to each other. In the word *washed*, spelling would suggest that the final sound of the word is that of *d*. If you say the word aloud, however, you'll find that the final sound is really that of *t*. Similarly, the sound of *sh* (/ʃ/ in IPA) occurs in both *shelf* and *tissue*. Even though the words are spelled differently, the actual speech sound produced is the same. Consequently, you may find yourself "unlearning" some spelling-reading listening habits that you have developed during your many years of primary and secondary schooling.

As you developed your understanding of oral language, you learned to recognize a finite number of different, recurring speech sounds that determine meaning. These are the **phonemes** of our language. You learned that English has consonant phonemes such as /p/ (*pie, open*) and /f/ (*four, telephone*). It also includes vowel phonemes such as /i/ (*eat, envy*) and /u/ (*tooth, dune*). Actually, these phonemes are abstractions rather than real sounds that occur. They are generalizations we make about a sound such as the /p/ phoneme. We place a phoneme in slash marks or **virgules** (/ /) when we are talking about the /p/ phoneme in general. However, the production of /p/ can vary, depending on its position in a word. In a word like *pie*, you hear audible aspiration (air release). You may or may not hear such aspiration in *hop*. Both these words contain variations, or **allophones**, of the phoneme /p/. To transcribe allophones, you will enclose the symbols in **brackets** ([ ]). When you transcribe actual speech, you should use brackets to enclose them. Such distinctions will become more clear as you learn IPA symbols and transcribe them.

The tables and figures on pages 2–4 are designed to serve as a reference for you as you complete Chapters 1–10. Table 1–1 and Figures 1–1 and 1–2 illustrate vowels and diphthongs according to pronunciation and formation. Tables 1–2 and 1–3 illustrate consonants according to pronunciation and place, manner, and voicing in production.

TABLE 1–1 INTERNATIONAL PHONETIC ALPHABET SYMBOLS: VOWELS AND DIPHTHONGS FOR MAINSTREAM AMERICAN ENGLISH[1]

Primary Orthographic Symbols	IPA Symbol	Key Words
ee	/i/	beet, meat
-i-	/ɪ/	bit, kiss
-e-	/ɛ/	bet, less
-a-	/æ/	bat, pass
-oo-	/u/	pool, too
-oo-	/ʊ/	book, could
-aw-	/ɔ/	saw, caught
-o-	/ɑ/	bond, odd
-ur-	/ɝ/	turn, earth, bird (stressed)
	/ɚ/	hamm<u>er</u>, und<u>er</u> (unstressed)
-u-	/ʌ/	up, come (stressed)
-u-	/ə/	el<u>e</u>ph<u>a</u>nt, b<u>a</u>nan<u>a</u> (unstressed)

TABLE 1–1 *(CONTINUED)*

Primary Orthographic Symbols	IPA Symbol	Key Words
a-e	/ɑ/	able, made, may (stressed)
a-e	/e/	vibrate, rotate (unstressed)
oa	/oʊ/	code, own, boat (stressed)
oa	/o/	disobey, rotation (unstressed)
i-e	/aɪ/	kite, ice, my
ou	/aʊ/	out, loud
oi	/ɔɪ/	coin, boy, oil

[1]Vowel symbols that are more characteristic of regional and cultural dialects will be introduced later in this book.

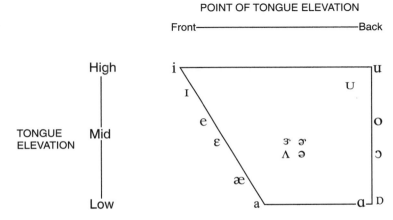

Figure 1–1 *Vowel sounds ordered by tongue elevation and position in the oral cavity. Adapted from the International Phonetic Association.*

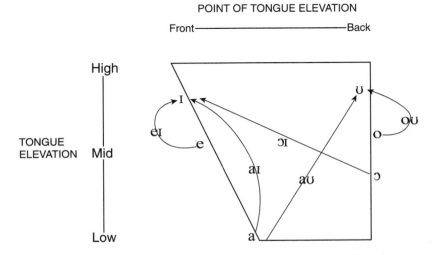

Figure 1–2 *Movement of rising diphthongs by tongue elevation and position in the oral cavity.*

TABLE 1–2 INTERNATIONAL PHONETIC ALPHABET SYMBOLS: CONSONANTS FOR
MAINSTREAM AMERICAN ENGLISH

Primary Orthographic Symbols	IPA Symbols	Key Words
p	/p/	pie, stopped, sip
b	/b/	boy, baby, cub
t	/t/	top, later, seat
d	/d/	down, ladder, red
k	/k/	come, baker, book
g	/g/	go, bigger, log
f	/f/	four, offer, calf
v	/v/	vine, over, believe
th	/θ/	thorn, nothing, earth
th	/ð/	them, bother, breathe
s	/s/	see, bicycle, ice
z	/z/	zoo, buzzer, eyes
sh	/ʃ/	shoe, mushroom, dish
zh	/ʒ/	measure, beige
h	/h/	hide, behind
ch	/tʃ/	chair, matches, such
j	/ʤ/	jump, angel, fudge
w	/w/	we, awake
y	/j/	yes, bayou
l	/l/	listen, hollow, fill
r	/r/	rain, arrange, car
m	/m/	me, omen, home
n	/n/	new, owner, pan
ng	/ŋ/	sing, singer

TABLE 1–3 CONSONANT SOUNDS OF AMERICAN ENGLISH BY PLACE AND MANNER
OF ARTICULATION

Manner of Production	Place of Articulation						
	Bilabial	Labio-dental	Lingua-dental	Lingua-alveolar	Lingua-palatal	Lingua-velar	Glottal
Stops	pb			td		kg	
Fricatives	ʍ	fv	θð	sz	ʃʒ	(ʍ)	h
Affricates					tʃ ʤ		
Nasals	m			n		ŋ	
Liquids				l	r		
Glides	w				j	(w)	

CHAPTER 1

PREPARATORY LISTENING EXERCISES

As you learned in Chapter 1 of your textbook, the relationship between phonemes and their orthographic representation can be highly variable. The following exercises are designed to help you develop your listening skills and decrease your reliance on visual orthographic symbols. USE THE INSTRUCTIONAL CD OR LISTEN TO YOUR INSTRUCTOR'S ORAL PRESENTATION TO COMPLETE THESE EXERCISES. Remember to focus on listening for phonemes, not spelling with letters.

A. CONSONANT EXERCISES

1. Orthographic consonant digraphs use two letters to stand for one phoneme. In the following words, circle each consonant digraph that actually is heard as a single phoneme. The first two have been marked to help you get started.

   (th)rew   ma(sh)   ba(th)e   fu(dg)e   ric(h)   han(g)
   bru(sh)   (ph)one   mo(th)   sin(g)s   bo(th)   (th)is

2. Two or more orthographic letters may be used to represent a single consonant phoneme. In the following words, circle the **two** consecutive consonants that represent a **single** consonant phoneme. The first two have been completed as examples.

   pe(pp)er   se(ss)ion   se(tt)ing   mu(tt)   ca(rr)y
   fa(ll)ing   hu(gg)ed   be(ll)   sli(pp)ed   mu(ff)

3. Orthography can also include letters for which there is no corresponding phoneme, that is, "silent" letters. In the following words, circle the letters that are silent, the ones that have no corresponding phoneme. The first two have already been completed to get you started.

   com(b)   (k)nife   (p)neumonia   (p)sychology   (g)nome
   (g)nat   (p)salm   paradi(g)m   autum(n)

4. Alphabetic letters do not always have a consistent one-to-one relationship with phonemes. In the following word lists, circle the **two** words that contain a **different** consonant phoneme than the other **four**, even though the spelling is the same for every word. Example a. has already been completed for you.

   a.   chew   chair   (chorus)   chin   china   (chic)
   b.   sugar   (lose)   insurance   conscious   ensure   (pose)
   c.   tragic   engine   (gang)   wager   (buggy)   giant

5. In this exercise, circle the **four** words in each line that contain the **same** phoneme, regardless of spelling. Then, using Table 1–2, determine which IPA symbol represents the sound common to the four words. The first two are done for you.

a.	(zebra)	(tons)	(whose)	azure	(busy)	hats	/z/
b.	(machine)	(ocean)	anchor	(shelf)	choose	(issue)	/ʃ/
c.	goat	(engine)	(joy)	(fudge)	(giant)	angle	/dʒ/
d.	aisle	(tax)	(scissors)	fusion	(racer)	(person)	/s/
e.	(young)	(few)	for	(William)	(onion)	funnel	/j/
f.	(who)	(high)	honest	weather	(ahead)	(whole)	/h/
g.	(trough)	(full)	(phone)	of	slough	(graph)	/f/
h.	(anger)	higher	rough	(grow)	(lager)	(pig)	/g/

B. Vowel Exercises

1. In orthographics, two or more letters can actually stand for only one vowel phoneme. In the following words, circle the **two** letters that correspond to only **one** phoneme. For example, *beat* has two vowel letters, *e* and *a*, but only one vowel phoneme, /i/. The first word has already been completed for you.

r(oa)d   (ou)tside   soupy   paid   c(oa)ster   m(ou)nded
br(oo)d   c(oi)led   r(ai)ning   vacation   racc(oo)n   b(oa)ting

2. Orthographics can also contain vowel letters for which there is no corresponding phoneme. In the following words, circle the letters that are silent. Note that the first word has already been completed as an example.

cod(e)   raged   fostered   troupe   etched   fume

3. Vowels used in word spelling do not necessarily correspond to the actual vowel represented. In each of the following lists of similarly spelled words, circle the word that has a vowel phoneme that is **different** from the other three words, even though all the words are spelled alike. Example a. has already been completed.

a.	down	(yellow)	Howard	clown
b.	shoe	poet	hoedown	floe
c.	meat	steam	bear	each

4. In contrast to the examples in exercise 3, words can share the same vowel phoneme but differ greatly in spelling. For the following word lists, circle the **four** words that have the **same** vowel phoneme. Then, using Table 1–1, find the IPA symbol representing that vowel. Again, the first two items are done for you.

a.	(rain)	(skein)	receive	(pane)	panic	(patriot)	/eɪ/
b.	(police)	(secret)	(peanuts)	vein	(beetle)	bread	/i/
c.	wrap	hot	sat	banana	mane	ashes	/ /
d.	book	hoop	grew	moose	flume	soot	/ /
e.	fad	possum	comb	pop	bond	soggy	/ /
f.	nut	ton	under	double	coupe	bonny	/ /
g.	bite	ravioli	bitter	rich	indigo	picture	/ /
h.	pout	wood	could	took	full	loop	/ /

5. Based on what you have learned in the previous exercises, determine the number of phonemes contained in each word. For example, the word *earth* contains

two phonemes /ɜθ/ but the word *fix* contains four phonemes /f ɪ k s/. Examples a. and b. have already been completed.

a. m /a/ tch /e/ s __5__   b. c /oa/ t/ _____3_____   c. find _____

d. summer _____   e. ink _____   f. kite _____

g. egg _____   h. speech _____   i. box _____

j. curve _____   k. tape _____   l. sun _____

6. For an extra challenge, try to reverse the phonemes in these words to make a new word; for example, *patch* becomes *chap* when its phonemes are reversed. Notice that the **spelling** can **change** but that the **phonemes** are the **same**. We've already done the first two for you.

a. choke ___c/oa/ch___   b. tube ___b/oo/t___   c. chirp _____

d. keys _____   e. lash _____   f. zoo _____

g. cub _____   h. I'd _____   i. scat _____

PART 2

TRANSCRIPTION OF VOWELS

CHAPTER 2

FRONT VOWELS
/i/ /ɪ/ /e/ /ɛ/ /æ/

As noted in Chapters 3 and 4 of the textbook, the nucleus of a syllable is usually a vowel. Vowels are characterized by closure of the velopharyngeal port, vocal fold vibration (voicing), and shaping of the oral cavity. The shaping of the oral cavity varies according to the location and height of tongue elevation. Traditionally, the front vowels are characterized by elevation of the front of the tongue toward the palate and alveolar ridge. The lips are unrounded and may be slightly retracted. As front tongue-to-palate distance changes, different vowels are produced. These changes in distance can be accomplished by tongue movement, jaw movement, or both. Five vowels are classified as front vowels: /i/ (as in *eat*), /ɪ/ as in *mitt*, /e/ as in *indicate*, /ɛ/ as in *bed*, and /æ/ as in *hat*. (Note that the diphthong /eɪ/ of stressed syllables occurs much more often than the monophthong /e/ of un-stressed syllables. See the textbook and Workbook Chapter 5, Vowels and Diph-thongs, for explanations and transcription exercises. In transcribing these vowels, the /i/ resembles a printed lowercase /i/, the /ɪ/ a miniaturized upper case I, the /e/ a lowercase *e*, the /ɛ/ a backwards 3, and the /æ/ the lowercase letters *a* and *e* made as a single, joined symbol. Actual front vowel pronunciation may vary across some dialects, but the reference dialect for these exercises is mainstream or general American English.

A. RECOGNITION

Listen to the instructional CD or to your instructor's live-voice presentation of List A. In each word list, there is one common front vowel phoneme. After listening to each list, fill in the IPA symbol for the common phoneme in the / / space at the top of the lists.

List 1 / ɪ /	List 2 / æ /	List 3 / i /	List 4 / ɛ /
lid	land	evil	bread
hymn	plaid	seam	ten
gym	have	bee	said
give	black	eat	guest
built	travel	these	leopard
business	latch	ski	ebb

List 5 / i /

busy
money
any
candy
dizzy
happy

List 6 / ɪ /

thinking
sink
being
going
baking
lacking

B. DISCRIMINATION

1. Listen to the instructional CD or to your instructor's live-voice presentation of Exercise B. In each list circle each word that contains the following:

List 1 /i/	List 2 /ɪ/	List 3 /e/	List 4 /ɛ/	List 5 /æ/
eve	myth	Kool-Aid	she	can
when	kitchen	indicate	hen	cane
tea	business	bear	red	calm
find	itched	alligator	belt	apple
chief	nylon	Patrick	friend	knack
rein	gym	enemy	many	call
marine	bitter	scarf	mean	half
style	sieve	renovate	men	backed
fish	lift	landscape	please	camera
demon	child	senator	eight	fade

2. Several of the front vowels are more variable in their pronunciation, depending on word context and the speaker's dialect. Listen for the vowels contrasts in the following word pairs.

a. /ɪ/   /ɛ/   b.   /ɪ/   /i/

tin	ten		it	eat
mitt	met		bin	bean
will	well		did	deed
bid	bed		mitt	meat
sit	set		pitch	peach

C. WORD TRANSCRIPTION FROM SPELLING/DICTATION

Listen to your instructor's presentation of the following word pair lists. Transcribe the front vowels heard.

EXERCISE 1: FRONT VOWEL CONTRAST DRILLS

List A: /i/–/ɪ/

1. least-list _/i/ - /ɪ/_

2. seep-sip _/i/ – /ɪ/_

3. lift-leafed _/ɪ/ - /i/_

List B: /i/–/ɛ/

1. lean-Len _/i/ /ɛ/_

2. met-meat _/ɛ/ /i/_

3. said-seed _/ɛ/ /i/_

List C: /ɪ/–/ɛ/

1. knit-net _____

2. wet-wit _____

3. lit-let _____

4. pit-Pete /ɪ/ /i/   4. Chet-cheat /ɛ/ /i/   4. beg-big _____

5. read-rid /i/ – /ɪ/   5. teen-ten /i/ /ɛ/   5. sit-set _____

6. feet-fit /i/ – /ɪ/   6. fell-feel /ɛ/ /i/   6. den-din _____

7. seen-sin /i/ – /ɪ/   7. lead-led /i/ /ɛ/   7. bed-bid _____

8. ship-sheep /ɪ/ – /i/   8. beast-best /i/ /ɛ/   8. will-well _____

List D: /ɛ/–/æ/

1. den-Dan _____

2. mess-mass _____

3. sad-said _____

4. Chet-chat _____

5. Ben-ban _____

6. pet-pat _____

7. fad-fed _____

8. tan-ten _____

List E: /æ/–/ɑ/

1. cat-cot _____

2. lap-lop _____

3. sod-sad _____

4. on-Ann _____

5. add-odd _____

6. pot-pat _____

7. psalm-Sam _____

8. rat-rot _____

EXERCISE 2: FRONT VOWELS

1. list _____

2. cap _____

3. dread _____

4. pony _____

5. eggs _____

6. sieve _____

7. gasp _____

8. seek _____

9. jest _____

10. risk _____

11. match _____

12. land _____

13. yeast _____

14. skip _____

15. etch _____

16. in _____

17. seat _____

18. rack _____

19. rich _____

20. shed _____

21. dream _____

22. jist _____

23. van _____

24. debt _____

25. ship _____

26. red _____

27. beech _____

28. catch _____

29. dent _____

30. feast _____

D. WORD TRANSCRIPTION FROM LIVE DICTATION

In this exercise, listen to the words presented and transcribe all the front vowels.

1. _____   11. _____

2. _____   12. _____

3. _____   13. _____

4. _____   14. _____

5. _____   15. _____

6. _____   16. _____

7. _____   17. _____

8. _____   18. _____

9. _____   19. _____

10. _____   20. _____

CHAPTER 3

BACK VOWELS

/u/ /ʊ/ /o/ /ɔ/ /ɑ/

Like the front vowels, the back vowels are also characterized by velopharyngeal closure, voicing, and varying degrees of tongue elevation. However, the distance between the palate and the back of the tongue (in contrast to the front of the tongue and the alveolar ridge for front vowels) increases as the speaker moves from the high back /u/ to the low back /ɑ/. These changes in distance can be accomplished by tongue movement, jaw movement, or both. Another contrast with front vowels is found in the lip shaping for /u/, /ʊ/ /o/, and /ɔ/: rounded and slightly protruded. Lip shaping for the /ɑ/ is simply open.

Five vowels are classified as back vowels: /u/ (as in *boot*), /ʊ/ as in *book*, monophthong /o/ as in *pianos*, /ɔ/ as in *law*, and /ɑ/ as in *lot*. In transcribing these vowels, the /u/ resembles a lowercase *u*, the /ʊ/ resembles an upside down omega, and the /o/, a lowercase *o*. The /ɔ/ resembles a backwards lowercase *c*, and /ɑ/ looks like the orthographic lowercase *a* (as opposed to a typeset *a*). (Note that diphthong /oʊ/ of stressed syllables occurs much more frequently than monophthong /o/ of unstressed syllables; see the text and Chapter 5, Diphthongs, in this workbook.) Actual back vowel pronunciation may vary across some dialects, especially for /ɔ/, but the reference dialect for the following exercises is mainstream American English.

A. RECOGNITION

Listen to the instructional CD or to your instructor's live-voice presentation of this exercise. In each word list, there is one back vowel phoneme common to the words. After listening to each list, fill in the IPA symbol for the common phoneme in the / / space provided at the top of the list.

List 1/ /	List 2 / /	List 3 / /	List 4 / /	List 5 / /
push	father	romantic	fruitful	awning
should	palm	cooperate	whose	audio
wool	knowledge	sailboat	crew	naught
book	cop	exponential	through	saw
good	honest	introduce	canoe	caught
wolf	bomb	oscilloscope	boot	thought

B. DISCRIMINATION

Listen to the instructional CD or to your instructor's live-voice presentation of this exercise. Circle each word that contains the following:

List 1 /u/	List 2 /ʊ/	List 3 /ɔ/	List 4 /ɑ/
tomb	wool	naught	common
stood	tool	pawnshop	honor
look	pool	call	alms
chewed	pull	shot	psalm
cruiser	hooked	hawk	father
blue	put	cot	gather
doom	but	bawl	auto
soup	good	ball	pawned
wood	full	caught	sob
cute	spook	got	oddity

C. WORD TRANSCRIPTION FROM SPELLING/DICTATION

Listen to your instructor's presentation of Lists A to C. Transcribe the vowels heard in each word pair.

EXERCISE 1: BACK VOWEL CONTRAST DRILLS

List A: /u/−/ʊ/	List B: /ɔ/−/ɑ/	List C: /ɑ/−/æ/
1. look-Luke _____	1. rah-raw _____	1. sod-sad _____
2. fool-full _____	2. sought-sot _____	2. lack-lock _____
3. who'd-hood _____	3. dawn-Don _____	3. sack-sock _____
4. soot-suit _____	4. caught-cot _____	4. Tom-tam _____
5. good-gooed _____	5. hock-hawk _____	5. hat-hot _____
6. kook-cook _____	6. Lon-lawn _____	6. chop-chap _____
7. pool-pull _____	7. awed-odd _____	7. ban-Bonn _____
8. stood-stewed _____	8. yon-yawn _____	8. gash-gosh _____

EXERCISE 2: BACK AND FRONT VOWELS

In this dictation exercise, transcribe both front and back vowels in the words dictated.

1. tools _____	7. eggnog _____	13. soot _____
2. bookshelf _____	8. shot _____	14. smoothly _____
3. logbook _____	9. castoff _____	15. thought _____
4. logic _____	10. pushing _____	16. ambush _____
5. popping _____	11. chops _____	17. fuse _____
6. costly _____	12. brooks _____	18. soup _____

19. baboons _____   23. sleuth _____   27. frost _____

20. pawned _____   24. cheesecloth _____   28. pulled _____

21. Polly _____   25. tossing _____   29. shop _____

22. shook _____   26. choose _____   30. holly _____

D. Word Transcription from Live Dictation

1. _____   11. _____

2. _____   12. _____

3. _____   13. _____

4. _____   14. _____

5. _____   15. _____

6. _____   16. _____

7. _____   17. _____

8. _____   18. _____

9. _____   19. _____

10. _____   20. _____

CHAPTER 4

CENTRAL VOWELS
/ɝ/ /ɚ/ /ʌ/ /ə/

As a class of vowels, the central vowels are all characterized by velopharyngeal closure, voicing, and varying degrees of tongue elevation. These vowels are produced with the tongue body varying in elevation in the center of the oral cavity. There is much less variation in tongue elevation for these vowels than for the front and back vowels, however. The /ɝ/ and /ɚ/ are produced with lip rounding, but not the /ʌ/ and /ə/. Furthermore, use of these vowels depends not only on the vowel sound but also on whether or not it is contained in an accented syllable. Four vowels are classified as central vowels, two stressed and two unstressed. /ɝ/ (as in *earth, burn*) and /ɚ/ (as in *mother, cover*) are the stressed and unstressed counterparts, respectively, for the *-er* vowel.

The vowel sound *-uh* is transcribed as /ʌ/ in stressed syllables (e.g., *mud, buggy*). The unstressed /ə/ (also known as schwa) is the last vowel in the word *panda* and the second vowel in the word *enemy*. To further clarify, the /ɝ/ and /ʌ/ symbols are used for syllables in which the *-er* or *-uh*, respectively, is accented (e.g., *turn, mug*). If a syllable with *-er* or *-uh* is unaccented, you will use the symbols /ɚ/ and /ə/, respectively, to transcribe them (e.g., *inner, atomic*). The /ɝ/ and /ʌ/ vowels are produced with more intensity and greater duration than their unstressed counterparts, /ɚ/ and /ə/. This means that you must pay attention not only to the **sound identity** of these vowels but also to their **syllable status** within a word. Additionally, **one-syllable** words with the *-er* or *-uh* vowel will always be transcribed with the **stressed** vowel symbols. As with previous drills, the reference dialect for the following exercises is mainstream (general) American English.

For Exercises A and B, listen to the presentations on the instructional CD or to your instructor's live-voice presentation.

A. RECOGNITION

In each word list, there is one central vowel phoneme common to all the words. After listening to each list, fill in the IPA symbol for the common phoneme in the / / space provided at the top of the list.

List 1 / /	List 2 / /	List 3 / /	List 4 / /
burning	luck	computer	alone
fern	usher	urbane	pigeon
merchant	oven	over	fountain
firm	jumped	labor	alphabet
learning	other	better	Alabama
worded	under	terrain	away

B. Discrimination

Listen to each word list and circle each word that contains the vowel phoneme at the top of the list.

List 1 /ʌ/	List 2 /ə/	List 3 /ɝ/	List 4 /ɚ/
full	diction	buzzer	supper
dull	awesome	fur	worse
ugly	upper	word	tailor
mother	banana	turned	pusher
put	tunnel	thorough	urban
come	begun	curried	burden
son	again	girl	zither
bush	lemon	offer	manner
fool	nothing	desert	nearer
does	attuned	dessert	cherry

C. Word Transcription from Spelling/Dictation

For Lists A and B, transcribe the central vowels heard in the word pairs. For Exercise 2, transcribe all front, back, and central vowels in the words dictated.

Exercise 1: Central Vowel Comparison Drills

List A: /ɝ/–/ɚ/

1. rooster _____

2. mermaid _____

3. earthy _____

4. purse _____

5. author _____

6. birds _____

7. murdered _____

8. nursery _____

9. Saturn _____

10. beginner _____

List B: /ʌ/–/ə/

1. rhumba _____

2. Russian _____

3. aluminum _____

4. guppy _____

5. mushroom _____

6. accomplish _____

7. police _____

8. sunny _____

9. even _____

10. aloof _____

Exercise 2: Front, Back, and Central Vowels

1. agriculture _____

2. meteor _____

3. Gertrude _____

4. reserve _____

5. earning _____   18. composer _____

6. slumber _____   19. version _____

7. helicopter _____   20. computer _____

8. earnings _____   21. shutter _____

9. thermos _____   22. chirped _____

10. thunder _____   23. touched _____

11. govern _____   24. kumquat _____

12. hamburger _____   25. buttercup _____

13. panther _____   26. snug _____

14. gazelle _____   27. thirsty _____

15. thumbtack _____   28. learning _____

16. crutch _____   29. turkey _____

17. enough _____   30. either _____

D. WORD TRANSCRIPTION FROM LIVE DICTATION

In this exercise, listen to all the words presented and transcribe all front, back, and central vowels.

1. _____   11. _____

2. _____   12. _____

3. _____   13. _____

4. _____   14. _____

5. _____   15. _____

6. _____   16. _____

7. _____   17. _____

8. _____   18. _____

9. _____   19. _____

10. _____   20. _____

DIPHTHONGS

Traditional/Rising: /eɪ/ /oʊ/ /aʊ/ /ɔɪ/ /aɪ/

Centering: /ɪɚ/ /ɛɚ/ /ɑɚ/ /ʊɚ/ /ɔɚ/

In contrast to the relatively fixed position of monophthong vowels, diphthongs are characterized by a transition from one vowel position to another in their formation. The tongue assumes the position for a monophthong vowel (onglide portion), but then moves quickly to another vowel position (offglide portion), so that only one sound is perceived.

There are several ways to classify diphthongs. The terms *rising* and *centering* refer to the direction of the tongue movement in the offglide portion. Thus, the rising diphthongs all end in a high front or back vowel, /ɪ/ or /ʊ/. The centering diphthongs all finish in a central vowel position, /ɚ/. Some phoneticians will simply transcribe /ɚ/-diphthongs as postvocalic consonant /ɹ/. Consequently, *car* could be transcribed as [k ɑ ɹ] or [k ɑɚ]. Another example would be transcribing *pear* as [p ɛ ɹ] or [p ɛɚ]. In this chapter, we will show you how to transcribe using /ɚ/-diphthongs. Later, in transcribing liquids (Chapter 10), we will again visit this topic.

The traditional, or rising, diphthongs constitute a much older classification grouping than the newer, centering, diphthongs. This is the reason they are often referred to as a "traditional" class. The /eɪ/ and /oʊ/ diphthongs are the stressed counterparts of the monophthongs /e/ and /o/. They are heard in words such as *lane* and *phone*. The /aʊ/ diphthong is heard in words such as *out, cow,* and *flounder*. /ɔɪ/ is found in words such as *boil, poignant,* and *coin*. Finally, /aɪ/ is heard in words such as *eye, piper,* and *height*. Regardless of the type of diphthong, be sure to connect the two vowel symbols when you transcribe diphthongs, or else use a ligature marking ([ɔɪ] to indicate that they constitute one diphthong, rather than two separate vowels i.e., [ɔ] and [ɪ]).

A. RECOGNITION

In each word list, there is one diphthong common to all the words. For each list listen to the words, then fill in the IPA symbol for the common phoneme in the / / space at the top of the list.

1. Rising Diphthongs

List A: / /	List B: / /	List C: / /	List D: / /	List E: / /
skate	cope	house	oyster	mighty
major	Polish	count	Polaroid	fine
sleigh	coat	crowd	foyer	sign
maniac	polar	loud	employ	china
caper	rose	down	moisture	tiger
danger	closing	pout	doily	riding

2. Centering Diphthongs

List A: / /	List B: / /	List C: / /	List D: / /	List E: / /
market	ear	pure	foreman	air
card	here	sure	chore	hare
heart	pier	pure	torn	share
carbon	steer	Murine	pouring	lair
scarred	cheer	curious	torso	barren
partake	mere	Puritan	corny	pear

B. DISCRIMINATION

Listen to the words in each list, then circle each word in the list that contains the diphthong indicated at the top of the list.

1. Rising Diphthongs

List A: /eɪ/	List B: /oʊ/	List C: /aʊ/	List D: /ɔɪ/	List E: /aɪ/
danger	hoping	count	poise	highly
prey	copy	foundry	porpoise	faithful
teak	doughnut	powder	hoist	kindness
eighty	loner	coach	mouth	binder
katydid	long	bower	boyish	minded
payment	coast	Maude	pause	rhinoceros
matinee	thrown	pouch	avoidance	child

2. Centering Diphthongs

List A: /ɔɚ/	List B: /ɪɚ/	List C: /ɛɚ/	List D: /ɑɚ/
hourly	fear	bear	hardest
courtship	bear	dark	partner
boarded	dear	airplane	Farsi
hoarse	sheer	mercy	gardener
border	near	careful	carrot
torch	church	rare	parsnip
curtain	gear	stairs	heartened
courtesy	hearing	stars	marvelous
scourge	herring	stirs	hare

In some dialects, the /ʊɚ/ diphthong may be produced as the central, stressed /ɝ/. Listen to the following contrasts between /ɝ/ and /ʊɚ/.

3. Contrasts: /ɝ/ and /ʊɚ/

/ʊɚ/	/ɝ/
pure	pure
purify	purify
sure	sure
Puritan	Puritan
Murine	Murine
cure	cure

C. WORD TRANSCRIPTION FROM SPELLING/DICTATION: ALL VOWELS AND RISING DIPHTHONGS

1. rhyme _____
2. chain _____
3. choice _____
4. high _____
5. rowdy _____
6. royalty _____
7. frown _____
8. training _____
9. somehow _____
10. polite _____

11. cape _____
12. coins _____
13. point _____
14. stage _____
15. only _____
16. station _____
17. couch _____
18. open _____
19. binder _____
20. praise _____

21. frowning _____
22. myself _____
23. joined _____
24. denounced _____
25. amaze _____
26. nineteen _____
27. housing _____
28. approach _____
29. reprise _____
30. founder _____

D. WORD TRANSCRIPTION FROM LIVE DICTATION

1. _____
2. _____
3. _____
4. _____
5. _____
6. _____
7. _____
8. _____
9. _____
10. _____

11. _____
12. _____
13. _____
14. _____
15. _____
16. _____
17. _____
18. _____
19. _____
20. _____

PART 3

TRANSCRIPTION OF CONSONANTS

CHAPTER 6

STOP CONSONANTS
/p/ /t/ /k/ /b/ /d/ /g/

We now turn to transcription of consonants. As noted in the textbook, consonants are not required for syllable formation, although English syllables commonly contain one or more consonants. They are characterized by resistance to the airstream. Consonants are classified according to place of articulation, manner of articulation, and voicing. We will present the consonants by manner category in this section of your workbook.

As a group, stops are characterized by an interruption of the voiced or voiceless airstream within the oral cavity, combined with velopharyngeal closure. Stops in American mainstream English are produced at three places of articulation: bilabial, alveolar, and velar. The stop consonants also occur in **cognate pairs** (same place and manner of articulation but differing in voicing). Cognates /p/ and /b/ are made with the lips closed. For cognates /t/ and /d/, the tongue tip closes against the alveolar ridge. Velar cognates /k/ and /g/ require the back tongue to be closed against the velum. Stops may or may not be released (produced with audible air release), depending on their position in the syllable and the consonants surrounding them. (We will cover aspiration and deaspiration in detail later in this workbook in Chapter 12). All the stop consonant symbols look very much like the lowercase alphabetic letters you learned to print when you began school. Note that the symbol for the velar /g/ appears like a hand-printed *g* rather than the typeset *g*.

A. RECOGNITION

In each word list, there is one common stop consonant. For each list listen to the words, then fill in the IPA symbol for the common phoneme in the / / space above the list.

List 1 / /	List 2 / /	List 3 / /	List 4 / /
clique	date	mattress	rabbit
park	today	taped	table
duck	waited	washed	tub
cloud	saved	debt	broad
ache	dressed	lettuce	number
occur	address	yacht	pebble

List 5 /   /   **List 6 /   /**
guest   placed
trigger   split
ghost   kept
rogue   pound
sag   keeper
eagle   happy

B. DISCRIMINATION

In each word list circle the words that contain the phoneme at the top of the list.

List 1 /p/	List 2 /b/	List 3 /t/	List 4 /d/	List 5 /k/	List 6 /g/
apple	rabbit	doubt	adore	rice	rough
spring	mob	Thomas	jumped	baroque	higher
psychic	thumb	laughed	medal	accord	again
hopped	absolved	math	Wednesday	church	finger
telephone	bomb	liked	should	chasm	ghost
paper	numb	ptomaine	middle	accident	example
staph	bright	antler	stopped	taxi	bragged
upon	ebony	ether	bathed	liquid	rogue

C. WORD TRANSCRIPTION FROM SPELLING/DICTATION: STOPS, VOWELS, AND DIPHTHONGS

1. paid _____

2. buggy _____

3. cub _____

4. god _____

5. candle _____

6. goody _____

7. gum _____

8. Gandalf _____

9. toad _____

10. teapot _____

11. dipped _____

12. kite _____

13. copay _____

14. bigot _____

15. pawed _____

16. dirt _____

17. bought _____

18. bandana _____

19. cutter _____

20. baton _____

21. pit _____

22. copy _____

23. get _____

24. gap _____

25. goad _____

26. biker _____

27. gab _____   29. cupcake _____

28. bad _____   30. decade _____

D. Word Transcription from Live Dictation: Stops, Vowels, and Diphthongs

1. _____   11. _____

2. _____   12. _____

3. _____   13. _____

4. _____   14. _____

5. _____   15. _____

6. _____   16. _____

7. _____   17. _____

8. _____   18. _____

9. _____   19. _____

10. _____   20. _____

FRICATIVES

Voiceless: /h/ /ʍ/ /f/ /θ/ /s/ /ʃ/

Voiced: /v/ /ð/ /z/ /ʒ/

The fricative consonant sounds are all characterized by continuous audible friction, which is caused by constriction in the oral cavity. Forcing air (voiced or unvoiced) through this constriction (a narrow opening) results in the airstream turbulence characteristic of fricatives. As with stop consonant formation, the velopharyngeal port is closed. English fricatives occur at five different places of articulation: labial, dental, alveolar, palatal, and glottal. Eight of the fricatives occur in cognate pairs: labiodental /f/ and /v/, dental /θ/ and /ð/, alveolar /s/ and /z/, and palatal /ʃ/ and /ʒ/. The glottal fricative, /h/, does not have a cognate. The bilabial fricative /ʍ/ (also sometimes transcribed as /hw/) is more often produced as the voiced glide /w/ in mainstream American English. Use of /ʍ/ in words such as *which* and *what* is generally typical of some regional dialects as well as the speech of older and more formal speakers of American English. Because /w/ is used much more often in mainstream American English, we will not transcribe /ʍ/ words here. (See Chapter 10, for /w/ transcription practice; Chapter 14, Changes in Voicing, includes transcription of /ʍ/).

Several of the fricative symbols are quite similar to printed letters; for example, /h/ resembles a printed lower case *h*, /f/ and /v/ look like printed *f* and *v*, respectively, and /s/ and /z/ can be written like lowercase *s* and *z*. The symbols for voiceless *th* (/θ/ in *thirteen, with*) and voiced *th* (/ð/ as in *them, breathe*) do not have similarly appearing alphabetic counterparts. The /θ/ symbol resembles a 0 (zero) with a line drawn across it. The /ʃ/ symbol (the phoneme heard in *shine* and *sure*) resembles an elongated sigmoid. The /ʒ/ symbol (the phoneme heard in *measure* and *leisure*) resembles a typeset *z* with a loop added to the bottom.

The following exercises are grouped separately in cognate pairs. Because there are so many fricatives, we felt that it would be helpful to limit the number in each presentation. The final dictation exercises will combine all the symbols.

1. EXERCISES FOR FRICATIVE COGNATE PAIRS: /f/–/v/ /θ/–/ð/ AND /h/

A. RECOGNITION

For each list, listen to all the words, then fill in the fricative symbol common to each list in the / / space at the top of the list.

List 1 / /	List 2 / /	List 3 / /	List 4 / /	List 5 / /
theirs	office	envy	faithful	behalf
weather	phonetics	of	fourth	heifer
neither	cough	heavy	birthday	hoof
southern	diphthong	leave	thresh	rehearse
breathe	half	marvel	health	whole
them	staff	vintage	arithmetic	high
bother	phase	move	moth	unholy
loathe	trough	pavement	anthem	behind

B. DISCRIMINATION

For each word list, listen to the words on the list, then circle the words containing the phoneme transcribed at the top of the list.

List 1 /f/	List 2 /v/	List 3 /θ/	List 4 /ð/	List 5 /h/
coffee	valet	these	these	honest
elephant	confusion	booth	they'll	who
fifteen	vacuum	thigh	weather	behind
prophet	driver	either	throw	half
half	offer	Thomas	bathe	hope
Steven	halves	hothouse	toothpaste	behave
fault	motherly	anthem	clothes	hour
infant	divide	south	heathen	backache
leaves	of	thorny	bathe	Ohio
farm	vase	myth	thyme	sigh

C. WORD TRANSCRIPTION FROM SPELLING/DICTATION: /f/–/v/ /θ/–/ð/ /h/

1. foot _____

2. eleventh _____

3. hopeful _____

4. teeth _____

5. vivid _____

6. fatherhood _____

7. breathe _____

8. froth _____

9. fate _____

10. heathen _____

11. birthday _____

12. beaver _____

13. pathway _____

14. fourth _____

15. victor _____

16. bother _____

17. thirty _____

18. huff _____

19. faith _____

20. they've _____

2. EXERCISES FOR FRICATIVE COGNATE PAIRS: /s/-/z/ /ʃ/-/ʒ/

A. RECOGNITION

For each word list, listen to the words, then fill in the fricative symbol common to each list in the / / space above the list.

List 1 / /	List 2 / /	List 3 / /	List 4 / /
treasure	zebra	nice	seashore
barrage	scissors	social	shares
azure	roses	police	partial
beige	ozone	precious	machine
measured	zealous	escape	portion
garage	please	mystery	sunshine
fusion	laser	size	lashes
corsage	lies	science	shoes

B. DISCRIMINATION

Listen to the following words, then circle the words that contain the phoneme indicated at the top of each list.

List 1 /s/	List 2 /z/	List 3 /ʃ/	List 4 /ʒ/
racer	enzyme	insurance	treasure
mouse	misery	pressure	confusion
icing	zigzag	occasion	ozone
escape	azure	confusion	beige
casual	rose	caution	position
tons	closure	washed	leisure
precious	visible	tissue	laser
feast	fused	leisure	anxious
ensure	clothes	lessen	usual
loose	leisure	fresh	casual

C. WORD TRANSCRIPTION FROM SPELLING/DICTATION: /s/-/z/ /ʃ/-/ ʒ /

1. sash _____
2. zookeeper _____
3. measured _____
4. seashell _____
5. azure _____
6. sheets _____
7. shoes _____
8. precious _____
9. pizza _____
10. treasured _____
11. Persia _____
12. wish _____
13. ozone _____
14. easier _____

15. pressure _____   18. seizure _____

16. pleasure _____   19. gazed _____

17. vicious _____   20. sister _____

D. WORD TRANSCRIPTION FROM LIVE DICTATION: FRICATIVES, STOPS, VOWELS, AND DIPHTHONGS

1. _____   11. _____

2. _____   12. _____

3. _____   13. _____

4. _____   14. _____

5. _____   15. _____

6. _____   16. _____

7. _____   17. _____

8. _____   18. _____

9. _____   19. _____

10. _____   20. _____

CHAPTER 8

AFFRICATES
/tʃ/ /dʒ/

The next manner of articulation you will learn is affricates. Affricates are characterized by a stoppage of the outgoing airstream, followed by a release with friction. Thus, they begin with oral cavity closure, like stops, but differ in the way they are released. The two American English affricates are cognates: voiceless /tʃ/ (as in *choice* and *watch*) and voiced /dʒ/ (as in *jump* and *ridge*). The /tʃ/ resembles a /t/ and /ʃ/ linked together, and the /dʒ/ looks like a linked /d/ and /ʒ/. Remember to make sure that the two parts of the symbol touch each other in transcription. Otherwise, your affricate transcription may be misinterpreted as two different phonemes, a stop and a fricative.

A. RECOGNITION

Listen to each list and fill in the common affricate symbol in the / / space at the top of each list.

List 1 / /	List 2 / /	List 3 / /	List 4 / /
judge	choose	champion	jar
ridge	watching	cheese	fudge
jester	anchovy	picture	badge
adjourn	china	reach	angel
pledge	fracture	catcher	cage
jump	future	latch	gentle

B. DISCRIMINATION

Listen to each of the word lists and circle the words that contain the affricate consonant transcribed at the top of each list.

List 1 /tʃ/	List 2 /dʒ/	List 3 /tʃ/	List 4 /dʒ/
scratch	large	chipmunk	jealous
choir	gopher	chorus	injure
natural	angel	backache	zoology
cheap	bungee	teacher	anger
Jeep	jealous	chain	ranger
capture	enjoy	charge	graduate
lecture	leisure	choral	linger
kitchen	etching	pitch	reached
catcher	larger	cache	brazier
wager	crutch	patch	engine

C. Word Transcription from Spelling/Dictation: Affricates, Fricatives, Stops, Vowels, and Diphthongs

1. stitches _____
2. dodge _____
3. childhood _____
4. chopsticks _____
5. trudging _____
6. subject _____
7. lodger _____
8. chives _____
9. overture _____
10. Jacob _____
11. patchwork _____
12. bandage _____
13. adventure _____
14. speech _____
15. theology _____

16. badge _____
17. scratched _____
18. cheek _____
19. jerked _____
20. tangerine _____
21. chased _____
22. french fries _____
23. cheesecake _____
24. cabbage _____
25. stretched _____
26. grudge _____
27. ventured _____
28. passenger _____
29. challenge _____
30. change _____

D. Word Transcription from Live Dictation: Affricates, Fricatives, Stops, Vowels, and Diphthongs

1. _____
2. _____
3. _____
4. _____
5. _____
6. _____
7. _____
8. _____
9. _____
10. _____

11. _____
12. _____
13. _____
14. _____
15. _____
16. _____
17. _____
18. _____
19. _____
20. _____

CHAPTER 9

NASALS
/m/ /n/ /ŋ/

The next manner class of consonant articulation, nasals, includes three consonant phonemes. Unlike other manners of consonant articulation, nasals are characterized by velopharyngeal opening, rather than closing. Because the velum is lowered, the voiced airstream is directed out through the nasal cavity rather than orally. Nasals are produced in three places of articulation: bilabial (/m/, as in *my, ham*), (lingua-)alveolar (/n/, as in *now, any*), and velar (/ŋ/, as in *sing, hang*). The /m/ resembles a printed lowercase *m*, and the /n/ has the appearance of a printed lowercase *n*. The symbol /ŋ/ begins like an *n* but is extended below the line and hooked slightly left. Unlike /m/ and /n/, /ŋ/ does not occur at the beginning of words in English.

A. RECOGNITION

Listen to the following word lists and fill in the nasal common consonant symbol in the / / space provided at the top of each list.

List 1 / /	List 2 / /	List 3 / /
nice	singer	hymn
end	bring	enemy
noise	anger	autumn
green	long	most
soon	language	lemming
any	mining	empty
knee	hanger	lamp
mnemonic	bank	plum

B. DISCRIMINATION

Listen to the word lists and circle the words containing the phoneme transcribed at the top of each list.

List 1 /m/	List 2 /n/	List 3 /ŋ/
calm	hymn	anxious
infamous	knob	angle
diaphragm	gnash	hinge
shined	reign	donkey

List 1 /m/	List 2 /n/	List 3 /ŋ/
summer	ink	branch
pneumonia	autumn	think
prism	gnat	song
mnemonic	bank	single
numb	cringe	singing

C. WORD TRANSCRIPTION FROM SPELLING/DICTATION: NASALS, AFFRICATES, STOPS, VOWELS, AND DIPHTHONGS

1. meter _____
2. gang _____
3. combing _____
4. remove _____
5. chimney _____
6. meant _____
7. infield _____
8. taking _____
9. singer _____
10. ones _____
11. drama _____
12. compete _____
13. sanding _____
14. smoking _____
15. hangers _____

16. himself _____
17. everything _____
18. sometimes _____
19. cantor _____
20. slingshot _____
21. stunning _____
22. nation _____
23. amend _____
24. pneumatic _____
25. smooth _____
26. then _____
27. longer _____
28. heading _____
29. motor _____
30. meaningful _____

D. WORD TRANSCRIPTION FROM LIVE DICTATION: NASALS, AFFRICATES, FRICATIVES, STOPS, VOWELS, AND DIPHTHONGS

1. _____
2. _____
3. _____
4. _____

5. _____
6. _____
7. _____
8. _____

9. _____   15. _____

10. _____   16. _____

11. _____   17. _____

12. _____   18. _____

13. _____   19. _____

14. _____   20. _____

ORAL RESONANT CONSONANTS
Glides and Liquids

GLIDES: /w/ /j/   LIQUIDS: /r/[1] /l/

The last manner category, oral resonant consonants (or approximants) actually can be subdivided into two smaller categories, liquids and glides. We include all four phonemes in one chapter for several reasons. First, the glides and liquids share a great deal in common, as you have discovered by reading about them in the textbook. Second, glides are frequently substituted for liquids in the speech of young children. It's not uncommon for a three-year-old to substitute a /j/ (as in *yes*) for the /l/ in *lemon*, resulting in [j ɛm ən]. Another common substitution in the speech of young children is replacing /r/ (as in *read*) with the glide /w/, producing [w i d]. All these consonants are characterized by alterations of resonating cavities, rather than friction or interruption of the oral airstream. For liquids, a fixed position is taken. Glides, however, are characterized by movement from a high vowel position (/i/ or /u/) to the vowel that follows. The IPA symbols for these phonemes look quite similar to their alphabetic printed counterparts, except for the symbol /j/. The phoneme /r/ in *ring* and *carry* looks like a printed lowercase *r*. Likewise, the /l/ in *lady* and *hello* resembles a printed lowercase *l*. The /w/ of *witch* and *west* looks just like a printed lowercase *w*. However, the phoneme /j/, which looks like a printed lowercase *j*, is the sound heard in words like *year* and *onion*. Refer to the textbook for more information on this consonant class.

A. RECOGNITION

In each word list there is one common glide or liquid. Listen to each word list, then fill in the IPA symbol for the common phoneme in the / / space provided at the top of each list.

List 1 / /	List 2 / /	List 3 / /	List 4 / /
listen	young	well	real
ally	foyer	lower	rewind
gold	music	sweep	royal
fuel	stallion	wind	train

---

[1]This symbol actually represents a trilled *r* whereas /ɹ/ represents American English consonant *r*. Because /ɹ/ is a recent IPA change and more difficult to transcribe, we use /r/ here. Follow your instructor's preference regarding this symbol.

List 1 / /	List 2 / /	List 3 / /	List 4 / /
swell	use	fewer	tomorrow
twelve	yo-yo	would	rayon
liberal	annual	towel	rowing

B. DISCRIMINATION

1. Listen to the word lists and circle the words that contain the phoneme at the top of each list.

List A: /w/	List B: /j/	List C: /l/	List D: /r/
reward	candy	gale	rhyme
memoirs	youthful	gulp	try
anywhere[2]	canyon	tulip	anchor
linguist	union	should	carrot
guide	booty	teller	bird
William	beauty	lilac	bread
watt	few	twelve	crowded
sword	yeast	would	rhythm
dwell	pewter	wall	Barry
shown	view	dearly	treasure

2. Consonant /r/ versus /ɚ/-diphthongs:
   a. The r-consonant that follows a vowel (postvocalic /r/) can be transcribed in one of two ways: as a consonant /r/ or as part of an /ɚ/-diphthong (see Workbook Chapter 5). Listen to the following words and transcribe each word with the consonant /r/ and then with the /ɚ/-diphthong. (The first two are done for you as examples.)

		/r/	**/ɚ/-diphthong**
1.	car	[kɑr]	[kɑɚ]
2.	bear	[bɛr]	[bɛɚ] or [bɛɚ]
3.	torn		
4.	fierce		
5.	party		
6.	yearly		
7.	morning		
8.	partake		
9.	dared		
10.	cheer		

---

[2]*Anywhere* may be produced with /w/ or /ʍ/, depending on speaker dialect and/or formality of speech.

b. It is important to distinguish the vowels /ɜ/ and /ɚ/ from the consonant singleton /r/. Listen to the following word lists and circle the words containing the phoneme indicated in the slash marks at the top of each list.

List 1 /r/	List 2 /ɚ/	List 3 /ɜ/	List 4 /r/
range	hammer	birch	trustee
earth	burden	standard	custard
butter	retry	crayon	broken
gray	dryer	turn	tearing
arrow	scary	murder	processor
prayer	understand	return	afraid
trailer	preacher	burn	courtesy
turn	overcoat	Barney	crowd
cream	mirthful	wordy	fur
frog	chair	corn	regal

c. The following words also demonstrate differences between the consonant /r/ and the /ɚ/ and /ɜ/ vowels. Listen to the following word pairs, and transcribe them. The first pair is done for you as an example. (Note that postvocalic /r/ is transcribed as consonant /r/, rather than as different /ɚ/-diphthongs.)

1. curtain ____[k ɜ t ə n]____   6. furnace _____

   carton ____[k ɑ r t ə n]____   fairness _____

2. hurry _____   7. firming _____

   Harry _____   farming _____

3. Carol _____   8. park _____

   curl _____   perk _____

4. furry _____   9. curb _____

   fairy _____   carob _____

5. hearts _____   10. worm _____

   hurts _____   warm _____

C. Word Transcription from Spelling/Dictation: All Consonants, Vowels, and Diphthongs

1. lodging _____   5. weakly _____

2. witch _____   6. cute _____

3. radar _____   7. laugh _____

4. lilac _____   8. valuable _____

9. yield _____   20. lacking _____

10. frog _____   21. youthful _____

11. freeway _____   22. yellow _____

12. water _____   23. cubic _____

13. relative _____   24. yarn _____

14. wishing _____   25. useful _____

15. towel _____   26. collar _____

16. proud _____   27. winter _____

17. future _____   28. sandwich _____

18. dwindle _____   29. woven _____

19. royal _____   30. react _____

D. Word Transcription from Live Dictation: All Consonants, Vowels, and Diphthongs

1. _____   11. _____

2. _____   12. _____

3. _____   13. _____

4. _____   14. _____

5. _____   15. _____

6. _____   16. _____

7. _____   17. _____

8. _____   18. _____

9. _____   19. _____

10. _____   20. _____

PART 4

USE OF NARROW TRANSCRIPTION SYMBOLS

As you read in the textbook in Chapter 6, phonemes produced in connected speech share overlapping coarticulatory movements. Consequently, phoneme identities can shift slightly or change completely, depending on their phonetic context. In this section, we give you opportunities to listen for, and practice, your narrow transcription skills. This means that you must be sensitive to allophonic variation and try to transcribe what you hear as accurately as possible. We will not cover all the IPA narrow transcription symbols in this section. We will give you practice in listening for allophonic variations and transcribing them accurately. We will cover the following diacritic markings in the next few chapters:

CHANGES IN DURATION

[ː]   indicates that a sound was unusually lengthened in duration.
       Example: same men [s e ɪ m ː ɛ n]
[ˌ]   indicates that a consonant has been given the duration of a syllable and is
       considered a **syllabic consonant.**
       Example: button [b ʌ t n̩]

ASPIRATION OF STOPS

[ʰ]   indicates that a stop consonant has been aspirated or audibly released.
       Example: pie [pʰ aɪ]
[̚]   indicates that a stop consonant was not aspirated or released.
       Example: up [ʌ p̚]

CHANGES IN PLACE

[̪]   indicates that an alveolar phoneme has shifted to a dental place of articulation
       due to influence of adjacent [θ] or [ð].
       Example: pass through [p æ s̪ θ r u]

CHANGES IN VOICING

[̬]   indicates that a sound that is usually voiceless is produced with voicing as a
       result of coarticulation.
       Example: birdhouse [b ɝ d h̬ aʊ s]
[̥]   Indicates that a consonant that is usually voiced was made without voicing.
       Example: play [p l̥ eɪ]

CHANGES IN RESONANCE

[˜]   indicates that a phoneme usually made with oral resonance is made with nasal resonance.

Example: moon [m ũ n]

CHAPTER 11

ALTERATIONS IN DURATION

We begin with those transcription symbols concerned with changes in the length of phonemes. The first symbol, [:], is applied when a vowel or a consonant is held slightly longer than usual. This symbol looks like a colon and immediately follows the phoneme that was lengthened. In transcription of normal, connected speech, it is most frequently used for phrases in which the first word ends in the same phoneme that begins the next word. Typically, you simply elongate the first sound in such cases rather than repeating the phoneme. For example, *some meat* becomes [s ʌ m: i t] rather than [sʌmmit]. *Same men* becomes [s eɪ m: ɛ n] rather than [s eɪ m m ɛ n]. (Note: We will discuss this effect on stops in Workbook Chapter 12, Aspiration of Stops.)

The second narrow transcription symbol of interest is the [ˌ], which is used to identify a **syllabic consonant**. Syllabic consonants are the only exception to the rule that says a syllable nucleus must be a vowel. The phonemes /m/, /n/, and /l/ can be lengthened to form an unaccented syllable when coarticulation makes a vowel unnecessary. Examples include *mitten* [mɪtn̩] as opposed to [mittɛn] and *candle* [k æ n d l̩] rather than [k æ ndʊ l].

Syllabic consonants most often result from two particular coarticulatory contexts. In one, the resonant consonant and the consonant preceding it share the same place of articulation (e.g., our examples of *mitten* and *candle*). In these cases, an intervening vowel is unnecessary because the tongue tip can maintain its alveolar position for both the phonemes. Thus, lengthening the [n] or [l] forms a syllable nucleus. The other context occurs when the articulators are free to move to the syllabic consonant while the preceding consonant is being made. Examples include *apple* [æ p l̩] and *driven* [d r ɪv n̩]. In these words, the alveolar position for [l] or [n] can be taken during production of the labial [p] or labiodental [v].

A number of syllabic consonants occur in rapid connected speech as a result of sound omissions and lengthening of [n] or [l]. We will give examples of these later in the workbook when we cover elisions/omissions (Chapter 15 in this workbook).

A. NARROW TRANSCRIPTION: LENGTHENING IN PHRASES

Listen to your instructor's presentation as you transcribe the following exercises. Transcribe the phrases in IPA symbols, and use the [:] symbol when applicable to indicate extended consonant duration.

Example: bus stop [b ʌ s: t ɑ p]

1. both thumbs _____   6. twelve vowels _____

2. bar rail _____   7. ban nukes _____

3. half full _____   8. same men _____

4. some mice _____   9. bathe them _____

5. call Linda _____   10. his zippers _____

B. NARROW TRANSCRIPTION: SYLLABIC CONSONANTS

Listen to your instructor's presentation of the following words. Each word will be presented twice, once with an intervening vowel and once with a syllabic consonant. The order of presentation will be varied. Determine which word (of the pair) contains the syllabic consonant. Transcribe the words in IPA symbols, and use the [ˌ] symbol to indicate syllabic consonant use. (Note: We have completed the first two examples for you.)

1. cattle	[k æ t ʊ l]	[k æ t l̩]
2. mitten	[m ɪ t n̩]	[m ɪ t ɛ n]
3. huddle	_____	_____
4. frozen	_____	_____
5. button	_____	_____
6. soften	_____	_____
7. bottle	_____	_____
8. hassle	_____	_____
9. topple	_____	_____
10. cable	_____	_____
11. ladle	_____	_____
12. sniffle	_____	_____
13. simple	_____	_____
14. satin	_____	_____
15. cotton	_____	_____

CHAPTER 12

ASPIRATION OF STOPS

You learned about aspiration of stops in Chapter 6 of the textbook. Now we will present exercises to help you develop your narrow transcription skills of this property. There are two symbols that you will learn to apply: [ʰ] for audible aspiration or audible stop release and [ˈ] when a stop is not audibly released. Remember, in English, prevocalic and intervocalic voiceless singleton stops are usually produced with audible aspiration. Final singleton stops may or may not be audibly released.

The presence of audible aspiration varies for consonant sequences containing stops. In general, these rules can be followed in transcription.

1. /s/ + stop prevocalic blends: stop will not be audibly released [ˈ].
   Example: spin [spˈɪn]

2. Nasal + stop postvocalic blends: stop will be audibly released.
   Examples: lamp [læmpʰ]   *sent* [sɛntʰ]   *sink* [sɪŋkʰ]

3. Fricative + stop postvocalic blends: stop will be audibly released.
   Examples: lisp [lɪspʰ]   *least* [listʰ]   *mosque* [mɑskʰ]

4. Postvocalic sequences composed of two stops: first stop will not be audibly released, but the second one will.
   Example: kept [kʰɛpˈtʰ]   *soaked* [s oʊkˈtʰ]

5. Intervocalic sequences composed of stops:
   a. If the stops differ in place of articulation, the first stop will not be audibly released, but the second one will.
      Example: potpie [pʰɑtˈpʰɑɪ]
   b. If the stops share place of articulation, the first stop will not be released and will be held longer than usual before the second stop is audibly released.
      Example: black cat [blækˈːʰæt]

See the textbook for further information about release and audible aspiration of stops.

A. NARROW TRANSCRIPTION OF SINGLETON STOPS

Listen to your instructor's presentation of the following words. Each word will be produced twice, with aspiration varying on the postvocalic stop. Insert [ʰ] and [ˈ] diacritic markings as appropriate. The first two are done for you.

1. pop   _____ [p ʰa p˺] _____   _____ [pʰ a pʰ] _____
2. type   _____ [tʰ aɪ pʰ] _____   _____ [tʰaɪp˺] _____

3. hat   _____   _____

4. seat   _____   _____

5. peek   _____   _____

6. loop   _____   _____

7. fought   _____   _____

8. bait   _____   _____

9. cot   _____   _____

10. cope   _____   _____

11. soap   _____   _____

12. shock   _____   _____

13. set   _____   _____

14. wrote   _____   _____

B. NARROW TRANSCRIPTION OF STOP SEQUENCES

Listen to your instructor's presentation of the following words. Review the rules on aspiration of stops in consonant sequences before you complete this exercise. The first two examples are completed for you.

1. kept _____ [kʰ ɛ p˺ tʰ] _____   11. hot tub _____

2. hot car _____ [hɑ t˺ kʰ ɑ r] _____   12. that car _____

3. laptop _____   13. into _____

4. daunt _____   14. sipped _____

5. lacked _____   15. can't _____

6. limp _____   16. that pair _____

7. sank _____   17. kicked _____

8. paste _____   18. camp _____

9. pine cone _____   19. wasp _____

10. leaked _____   20. missed _____

C. NARROW TRANSCRIPTION OF STOPS: SINGLETONS AND SEQUENCES

Listen to your instructor's presentation of the following words. Transcribe stops using [ʰ] or [ˀ] appropriately.

1. acorn _____

2. cake _____

3. back porch _____

4. hopping _____

5. payment _____

6. coattails _____

7. spurt _____

8. stuck _____

9. last _____

10. pop-top _____

11. apple _____

12. skip _____

13. recover _____

14. popcorn _____

15. cusp _____

16. rent _____

17. take care _____

18. short _____

19. laughed _____

20. puppy _____

CHAPTER 13

ASSIMILATORY CHANGES
Place and Resonance

In Chapter 6 of the textbook, you learned how consonant place of articulation may shift in rapid connected speech. Alveolar consonants /t d s z n l/ become dentalized if they occur next to an interdental [θ] or [ð]: *one thing* [w ʌ n̪ θ ɪ ŋ]. In phrases such as *Ridge Street*, the [s] will often shift to palatal [ʃ] as a result of assimilation: [r ɪ ʤ ʃ t r i t]. Such place shifts allow more rapid coarticulation movements and contribute to the smooth flow of speech. The following exercises are designed to help you recognize and correctly transcribe such place shifts. We have completed the first two examples for you in each exercise.

A. DENTALIZATION

1. one thumb _____ [w ʌ n̪ θ ʌ m] _____

2. both ties _____ [b o ʊ θ t̪ aɪ z] _____

3. code them _____

4. eighth star _____

5. with Tom _____

6. moth trap _____

7. bath soap _____

8. ride there _____

9. in there _____

10. cloth towel _____

11. lose them _____

12. south toll _____

13. on this _____

14. even though _____

15. fourth time _____

16. health text _____

B. OTHER ASSIMILATORY PLACE SHIFTS

1. place shift _____ [p l eɪʃ : ɪ ft] _____

2. miss Sheila _____ [m ɪ ʃ : i l ə] _____

3. Pat's chalk _____

4. mouse cheese _____

5. Bench Street _____

6. fudge sundae _____

7. porch swing _____

8. loose shelf _____

9. glass shop _____

10. bass shop _____

C. Assimilation Nasality

Chapter 6 in the textbook also introduced you to the effect of nasal consonants on vowels in rapid connected speech. Especially when a vowel comes between two nasal consonants or is a word-ending vowel following a nasal consonant, there will be a nasal resonant quality to the vowel. The diacritic marking [˜] is used to transcribe this **assimilation nasality.**

1. banana _____[b ə n æ̃ n ə̃]_____   7. meantime _____

2. monk _____[m ʌ̃ ŋ k]_____   8. hammer _____

3. mention _____   9. honey _____

4. framing _____   10. mommy _____

5. number _____   11. known _____

6. meaning _____   12. monkey _____

D. Combined Exercise

Now, put together what you have learned in this chapter about assimilation changes and use phonetic (narrow) transcription for the following words:

1. nine things _____[n ãɪ n̪θɪ ŋz]_____   8. with Nan _____

2. fourth morning _____[fɔrθmɔ̃r n ĩ ŋ]_____   9. pass Chinese _____

3. glass shelf _____   10. morning anthem _____

4. glass ship _____   11. Minnie Mouse _____

5. mention them _____   12. has shoes _____

6. loose change _____   13. eat there _____

7. mourned them _____   14. main theme _____

CHAPTER 14

CHANGES IN VOICING

Another characteristic of connected speech discussed in Chapter 6 of the textbook concerns changes that can occur in voicing as a result of coarticulation. Although you learned that vowels and certain consonants are always voiced whereas other consonants are voiceless, these properties can shift within connected speech. If there is a total voicing change and the affected consonant has a cognate, then the cognate will be transcribed. For example, the word *butter* could be transcribed as [b ʌ t ɚ] or [b ʌ d ɚ], depending on the amount of voicing of the intervocalic alveolar stop.

However, cognates are not available for liquids, glides, and the glottal voiceless fricative /h/. Consequently, you must use diacritic markings to indicate voicing changes for these phonemes. Narrow transcription uses the symbol [̥] (resembling a small *o*) beneath the affected phoneme to indicate devoicing. Liquids and glides will be devoiced when they occur in a blend following a voiceless fricative or stop. Examples of this occur in words like *shrimp* [ʃɹ̥ɪmp] and *cute* [k j u t]. In words with /s/ + /w/ blends, the actual phoneme used may be the voiceless /ʍ/: *sweet* [sʍit] and *swim* [sʍɪm]. Such devoicing will not occur in a three-element blend such as -*spl* or -*skr*. The addition of /s/ greatly reduces the audible release of the second, voiceless consonant so that [̥] is not needed. Note the difference in narrow transcription for these two words: *slat* [slæt] and *splat* [spl̥æt].

You also read in the text about a voicing change called **intervocalic voicing.** Intervocalic voiceless singleton consonants are particularly subject to this effect, especially /h/ and /t/. Quite often, intervocalic /t/ is heard with partial voicing in words like [bnt̬ɚ] or as its voiced cognate in words like *matter* [m æ d ɚ] and *otter* [ɑ d ɚ]. Because /h/ has no cognate, intervocalic voicing of this fricative must be indicated by the narrow transcription symbol [̬]. Consequently, correct narrow transcription of *birdhouse* would be [b ɝ d ḫaʊ s].

The exercise on the next page is designed to help you recognize and transcribe changes in voicing. We have completed the first two items as examples.

A. NARROW TRANSCRIPTION: VOICING CHANGES

1. plate _____ [p l̥ eɪ t] _____
2. three _____ [θ ɹ̥ i] _____
3. stagehand _____
4. behind _____
5. sleepy _____
6. club _____

7. pressure _____

8. bitter _____

9. cucumber _____

10. cluster _____

11. litter _____

12. cracker _____

13. row house _____

14. frayed _____

15. rehearse _____

16. please _____

17. Cuba _____

18. atrium _____

19. motor _____

20. feud _____

CHAPTER 15

ELISION/OMISSION AND ADDITION/EPENTHESIS

The demands of coarticulation in connected speech can also result in omission or addition of a phoneme or phonemes, as explained in Chapter 6 of the textbook. Sometimes, the demands of connected speech lead to the loss of whole syllables, particularly unaccented ones. Such elision or omission is typically seen in the rapid coarticulation of expressions such as *meat and potatoes* as [m i t n̩ p ə t eɪ t o z].

A. SYLLABLE OMISSION

Transcribe in IPA symbols each of the following words in two ways: first with "careful" pronunciation and second with natural, "casual" pronunciation typical of word production in a sentence. Pay special attention to the underlined syllables. The first example is done for you.

	Careful	Casual
1. vete_ran	[v ɛ t ɚə n]	[v ɛ t r ə n]
2. nati_onal		
3. int_erest		
4. choc_olate		
5. vege_table		
6. fed_eral		
7. reas_onable		
8. fav_orite		
9. sep_arate		
10. temp_erature		

B. EPENTHESIS

Other demands of coarticulation result in the insertion of a glottal stop [ʔ] (resembling a question mark without a dot) or an "intrusive" [w] or [j]. Less commonly, an intrusive /p/, /t/, or /k/ may occur in certain coarticulatory environments.

We'll begin with the phonetic environments for /w/, /j/, and /ʔ/ because they often occur under similar circumstances. Most often, when one syllable ends in a vowel and the following syllable begins in a vowel, some type of intruded consonant or /ʔ/ is necessary to distinguish between the two different vowels and establish that there are two syllables rather than one. For example, in the phrase *he eats*, a palatal /j/ or glottal /ʔ/ will intrude, [h i j i t s] or [h i ʔ i t s]. These additions signal to the listener that two words are present, rather than the single word *heats* [h i t s]. The glide /j/ typically intrudes after /I/ or /i/, whereas the /w/ follows /u/ or /ʊ/. An intruded glide or glottal stop /ʔ/ may also occur after diphthongs. Speakers can differ in the force with which they produce these intruded sounds. See Chapter 6 in the textbook for more information and examples of epenthesis.

/w/ /j/ /ʔ/

Transcribe in IPA symbols the following phrases, treating each group of words as a single speech utterance. In the first column, insert /w/ or /j/ as appropriate. In the second column, insert a glottal stop. The first example is done for you.

	Intrusive Glide	Glottal Stop
1. be evil	[b i j i v l̩]	[b i ʔ i v l̩]
2. go out		
3. see it		
4. stay in		
5. how are		
6. sue us		
7. new ale		
8. tie up		
9. two apples		
10. you all		
11. we each		
12. too easy		
13. he always		
14. who else		
15. may also		

The other commonly occurring example of epenthesis is found when nasals /m/, /n/, or /ŋ/ are followed by a voiceless fricative, as in words like *hamster, dance,* and *length.* As pressure builds up for the fricative following the nasal /m/, /n/, or /ŋ/, a voiceless stop may result, for example, [h æ m p s t ɚ], [tʃ æ n t s], and [l ɛ ŋ k θ]. The stop that intrudes is always in the same place of articulation as the nasal. This third exercise is designed to give you practice in detecting these intrusive stops.

NASALS + INTRUSIVE STOPS

All of the following words end in a nasal + fricative sequence, making them susceptible to stop intrusion. Fill in the appropriate intrusive stop. We have completed the first two as examples for you.

1. warmth _____ [w ɔ r m p θ]   6. prince _____

2. once _____ [w ʌ n t s]   7. answer _____

3. hamster _____   8. emphasis _____

4. tenth _____   9. cancel _____

5. strength _____   10. length _____

PART 5

MARKINGS FOR SPEECH RHYTHM

CHAPTER 16

ACCENT

Chapter 6 in the textbook introduces you to the concepts of speech rhythm, accent, and stress. In this chapter, we include practice for assigning **accent**, the stress placed on a syllable within a word. Remember that a syllable has a single vowel, diphthong, or syllabic consonant as its nucleus. The number of consonants in a syllable can vary, but more than one vowel means that you have more than one syllable. Thus, *stretched* [str ɛ ʧ t] (five consonants but one vowel) consists of only one syllable, but *eon* [i j ɑ n] or [iʔɑ n] is two syllables.

Also in Chapter 6 of the textbook, you learned that for every English word, one syllable will be stressed above the others. These stressed syllables will be audibly different from those with less stress: louder, longer, and slightly higher in pitch. American English has three relative accent levels that influence transcription: primary accent, secondary accent, and unaccented. (More levels may be identified, but we will confine ourselves to these three in these exercises.) Actual assignment of accent in American English is mostly a matter of conventional usage rather than a few standard rules.

We will follow IPA conventions in this chapter for marking accent. You will mark a syllable with primary accent by placing a dark, vertical line above and to the left of the affected syllable. For syllables with secondary accent, place a vertical line below and to the left of the affected syllable. Unaccented syllables remain unmarked, and their vowel nucleus is usually an /ə/. Thus, in the word *listen*, accent would be marked as follows: [ˈl ɪ s n̩]. In the three-syllable word *celebrate*, you would add these markings for accent: [ˈs ɛ l ə ˌb r e t]. In compound words like *football*, the syllables receive almost equal stress, so that no syllable is unaccented: [ˈf ʊ t ˌb ɔ l].

For further information on accent and changes in vowel pronunciation, see your textbook, Chapter 6. The following exercises on the next page are designed to help you listen for, and transcribe, varying levels of accent. In each exercise, we have completed an example for you to get you started.

A. DISCRIMINATION

Circle each word that contains:

1. 2 Syllables
   accent
   backed
   boa
   tearing
   very
   loaded
   splashed
   diphthongs
   kitten
   aversion

2. 1 Syllable
   based
   snows
   kicked
   tasted
   dried
   coded
   drowned
   borne
   little
   branched

3. 5 Syllables
   reactionary
   disability
   misarticulated
   pronunciation
   inspiration
   analysis
   laryngology
   velopharynx
   maladjusted
   unreality

4. 4 Syllables
   dictionary
   primarily
   description
   unaccented
   substitute
   approximate
   consonants
   continuation
   exhalation

5. 3 Syllables
   construction
   amazed
   checkered
   syllable
   nucleus
   combination
   primary
   information
   coriander

B. WORD TRANSCRIPTION

Listen to your instructor pronounce the following words. Include marks for primary accent and secondary accent. Unaccented syllables should be unmarked and contain /ə/ as their syllable nucleus.

1. observed _____ [əbˈz ɝ vd]_____

2. cattle _____ [ˈk æt̬ l̩]_____

3. ornament _____

4. friction _____

5. gigantic _____

6. telephone _____

7. riding _____

8. computer _____

9. fellow _____

10. psychology _____

11. reminded _____

12. indicate _____

13. appeared _____

14. character _____

15. pounding _____

16. language _____

17. standard _____

18. xylophone _____

19. joyfully _____

20. exclamation _____

21. gently _____   26. television _____

22. digital _____   27. mystery _____

23. nasality _____   28. hamburger _____

24. muffler _____   29. phonetics _____

25. liberal _____   30. conservative _____

CHAPTER 17

EMPHASIS AND INTONATION

Emphasis is the stress placed on a word within a phrase or a sentence. The words you emphasize in an utterance will be determined by your communicative intent, not by convention (as accent is). You may choose to emphasize one, two, or several words in a phrase. Short connecting words such as *a, the, of, and, some, or,* and *for* are seldom emphasized unless you have a particular reason to do so, for example, "a government *of* the people, *by* the people, and *for* the people." If a speaker emphasizes a word by producing it with greater force, it may be marked by underlining it. Double underlining can be used for very heavy emphasis. You may draw these emphasis lines under either regular spelling or IPA transcription.

Emphasis is used to focus the listener's attention on important words. You might emphasize a single word for identification, as in "Her car is a Beetle" or "She is studying audiology." You may also use emphasis of key words in parallel phrases to help your listener make a comparison: "We came early and left early" or "We came early and left late." You may also use emphasis in response to a specific question. "It was a big gray cat" would be the right emphasis if someone had asked you about the size of the animal. You may find further information about emphasis in the textbook in Chapter 6.

A. RECOGNITION

Read the following sentences aloud, observing the emphasized words. Try to imagine the situation for which each sentence would be appropriate.

1. That baby is crying again.   4. That baby is crying again.
2. That baby is crying again.   5. That baby is crying again.
3. That baby is crying again.   6. That baby is crying again.

B. DISCRIMINATION

For the sentences on the next page, connect each statement on the left with the appropriate question on the right by drawing a line between them. We have already completed the first example for you.

1. He saw a big red bird.   Did he see two big red birds?
2. He saw a big red bird.   Was the big bird he saw red or blue?
3. He saw a big red bird.   What was that big red animal he saw?
4. He saw a big red bird.   Who saw a big red bird?
5. He saw a big red bird.   Did he see a little red bird?
6. He saw a big red bird.   Are you sure a big red bird was there?

C. Transcription

Underline the words most likely to be emphasized in the following sentences to help a listener compare key words. We have completed the first example for you.

1. We <u>did</u> it, but we didn't <u>want</u> to.
2. They arrived, and then we arrived.
3. We drove home, but they walked home.
4. They went on a bus, and we went on a train.
5. A thesaurus is like a dictionary.
6. A penny saved is a penny earned.
7. We came early, and they came late.
8. I came, I saw, I conquered.
9. The spirit is willing, but the flesh is weak.
10. He said yes, but he meant no.

Intonation refers to the pattern of change in your fundamental voice pitch during a phrase. This rising and falling pitch is sometimes called **inflection**. Like emphasis, your use of intonation provides a level of meaning over and above the string of phonemes and the pattern of accent. Four pitch relative levels are commonly recognized in mainstream American English intonation. Level 2 is considered the standard, or baseline, from which your pitch rises to 3 or falls to 1. Level 4 is used only for expressions of surprise and high emotional outbursts. The direction of pitch change is more significant than the relative level in conveying meaning, however. The following example shows markings for both relative pitch levels and intonation contours:

$$\text{3} \qquad\qquad \text{3}$$
$$\underline{\text{Hurry up!}} \qquad \text{He's coming.}$$
$$\text{2} \qquad\qquad \text{2}$$

The next example shows the fourth relative level typical of surprised exclamation:

$$\text{4}$$
$$\text{My goodness!}$$
$$\text{2} \qquad \text{2}$$

Fortunately, for most purposes, it will be sufficient to mark intonation by using the connected contour lines, with sloping to indicate rate of change. You may use these contours with either regular word spelling or IPA transcription. When a continuous intonation contour is associated with regular spelling, it can reflect the length of a speech phrase. Note the following example:

The bus has left.   Left!   It's not fair.

Intonation tells your listener something special about your message. It interacts with emphasis to help stress key words. It may also indicate whether an utterance was a statement or a question. In its simplest forms, a rising intonation contour "mmmmm" [m : : :] indicates a question, whereas a falling contour on the same sound indicates the conclusion of a statement. You may also use a rising intonation contour to tell your listener, "There's more to come." Notice how this affects the following example:

We eat with knives, forks, and spoons.

Intonation can vary for questions, depending on the type of answer required. For example, yes-no questions usually have a rising intonation contour at the end. *Wh*-questions (*who, what, when, where, why*) typically rise and then fall. Notice these examples:

Is this the time?

When do you want to go?

D. MARKING INTONATION CONTOURS

Using contour lines, mark the appropriate intonation patterns for the sentences on the next page. We have completed the first sentence for you as an example.

1. Is this really the place?
2. They brought pretzels, hot dogs, potato chips, and beer.
3. Good morning. Is it time to go?
4. How many cookies do you want?
5. We're coming! We're coming! Wait a minute.
6. Mmmmmm, that's good.
7. Section thirteen is about computers.
8. Here today, gone tomorrow.
9. He said he was going where?
10. I guess that's the end of the chapter.

CHAPTER 18

TRANSCRIPTION OF CONNECTED SPEECH

Although you read and write distinctly separated word units, you produce and hear spoken language in uninterrupted phrases of coarticulated phonemes. Word boundaries are not apparent in these speech phrases, but you infer them from your knowledge of the language. To accurately transcribe connected speech, you should group phonemes into phrases, regardless of word boundaries.

So far in this workbook you have maintained word boundaries in IPA transcription. This practice can be misleading when we consider the nature of real connected speech. It overlooks the coarticulation effects where two words usually join. For example, two of the same adjoining sounds may become one phoneme, as in *some milk* [s ʌ m : ɪ l k]. Similar sounds may actually be omitted. Examples are found in the phrases *have fun*, which may be coarticulated as [h æ f : ʌ n], and *as soon*, produced as [æ s: u n]. /h/ and /ð/ are often omitted in connected speech, for example, *where is he* as [w ɛ r ɪ z i] and *who's that?* as [h u z æ t].

When you transcribe phonemes into larger visibly connected speech units, you also define the phrasing and pauses of natural flowing speech. This can reflect the rhythm of a person's speech pattern or dialect area. Transcription of connected speech requires you to forget word boundaries and listen instead for silent intervals that signal pauses. The spaces between coarticulated phones should be closer than the spaces between separated phrases.

You do not need to use written punctuation (e.g., periods, commas, and question marks) when you are transcribing connected speech. If punctuation marks will help a reader understand meaning, you should place them outside the square brackets. Because you are transcribing in the IPA, you do not use any capitalization. Furthermore, in purely phonetic transcription, pauses and speech phrases are the only appropriate punctuation.

When you read IPA transcription of connected speech, you must call up the auditory image of units of speech. You may have to repeat a phrase several times to determine the words and consequent meaning.

PHRASE AND SENTENCE RECOGNITION

Read each of the following phrases and sentences to determine their meaning. Transliterate (write orthographically) your interpretation on the adjoining line. Then circle the places in which coarticulation of adjoining words has influenced phonetic transcription. We have completed the first sentence for you as an example.

1. [ˈw ɛ r i ˈg o ʊ ʔ n̩] _____ Where's he going? _____

2. [aɪ d l aɪk ə bɝgɚ n̩ fr aɪ z] _____

3. [aɪsɔsəm:ɪ l k n̩ ə f r ɪ ʤ] _____

4. [w ɛ n l̩ i k ʌ m] _____

5. [wiʔ eɪ t m i t n̩ p ə t eɪ t əz f ɚ d ɪ n ɚ] _____

_____

6. [ɪ t h æ p n̩ d a n ə f ɔ r θ ə ʤ ə l aɪ] _____

_____

7. [ɪ z: æ t ə n u h æ t] _____

8. [aɪ w ɑ n ʧ ə t ə k ʌ m ɪ n s aɪ d] _____

_____

9. [h u z i k ɪ d n̩] _____

10. [h a ʊ m̩ aɪ d u n̩] _____

11. [w ɛ n z i l i v n̩] _____

12. [d ɪ ʤ ə w ɑ n f r aɪ z w ɪ ð æ t] _____

_____

13. [b ɪ z i æ z ə b i] _____

14. [w ʌ z i k ʌ m n̩ b aɪ tr eɪ n ɚ b ʌ s] _____

_____

15. [aɪ w ɑ n ə p i t z ə w ɪ ð e v r i θ ɪ ŋ] _____

_____

PART 6

DIALECTIC VARIATIONS

CHAPTER 19

DIALECTS AND /ɹ/ /ɝ/ /ɜ/ /ɚ/

American English pronunciation includes a number of dialects that are geographic, social, and/or ethnic in origin. A dialect is defined as a form of a language that is associated with one or more of these factors. Despite some possible phonological, morphological, and syntactic differences, a dialect shares many characteristics with the mainstream language. You will find a review of both major regional and cultural dialects of the United States in Chapter 8 of the textbook.

Up to this point, our frame of reference for transcription has been mainstream American English. However, there are other phonemes that occur in certain dialects of American English that we have not yet covered. One of these is the /ɜ/, which is most often used in New England, the Middle Atlantic seaboard, and the Southeast. (It looks rather like a miniaturized 3.) Its use corresponds to that of /ɝ/ in other American English dialects. If you are used to producing /ɝ/ in your speech, try this positioning to produce /ɜ/: put your tongue in the position you would use to produce the /ɝ/, but have the tip of your tongue placed against the lower front teeth. You can also produce /ɜ/ by beginning with the /ʊ/ tongue position, then raising the front portion of your tongue slightly, but leaving the tip against the front teeth.

A. PRODUCTION AND RECOGNITION

Try producing the following words first with the [ɝ] and then with [ɜ], feeling the tongue positions. If you are a native speaker of [ɜ], practice the exercise in the opposite order.

1. sir   [s ɝ]   [s ɜ]
2. work   [w ɝ k]   [w ɜ k]
3. curb   [k ɝ b]   [k ɜ b]
4. dirt   [d ɝ t]   [d ɜ t]
5. thirsty   [θ ɝ s t i]   [θ ɜ s t i]
6. deserve   [d ɪ z ɝ v]   [d ɪ z ɜ v]

You learned earlier that the unstressed /ɚ/ corresponds to the stressed /ɝ/ in mainstream American English. In dialects that use the /ɜ/, the unstressed counterpart is transcribed as /ə/. Try practicing these vowel sounds in the following words.

7. worker [w ɝ k ɚ] [w ɜ k ə]
8. earnest [ɝ n ə s t] [ɜ n ə s t]
9. bigger [b ɪ g ɚ] [b ɪ g ə]
10. burner [b ɝ n ɚ] [b ɜ n ə]
11. prefer [p r ɪ f ɝ] [p r ɪ f ɜ]
12. urbane [ɚ b eɪ n] [ə b eɪ n]

B. DISCRIMINATION

It may help you to discriminate and produce the /ɜ/ if you compare it to other vowels with which it can be confused: /ʌ/ and /ʊ/. Practice producing the following words, and, if possible, have a native user of /ɜ/ produce the words as you listen and transcribe them.

1. lurk [l ɝ k]   2. pert [p ɝ t]   3. curd [k ɝd]   4. purse [p ɝs]
   luck [l ʌ k]   putt [p ʌ t]   cud [k ʌ d]   pus [p ʌs]
   lurk [l ɜ k]   pert [p ɜ t]   curd [k ɜ d]   purse [p ɜs]
   look [l ʊ k]   put [p ʊ t]   could [k ʊ d]   puss [p ʊ s]

C. WORD TRANSCRIPTION FROM SPELLING/DICTATION

You may complete this exercise by pronouncing and transcribing these words yourself, or you may listen to your instructor's dictation of the words. If you are a native speaker of /ɝ/ and /ɚ/, transcribe the words using /ɜ/ and /ə/, then pronounce each word after you transcribe it. If you are a native user of /ɜ/ and /ə/, however, transcribe and pronounce the words using /ɝ/ and /ɚ/ instead.

1. sermon _____   6. after _____

2. avert _____   7. learner _____

3. desert _____   8. shirker _____

4. dessert _____   9. water _____

5. furnace _____   10. eastern _____

Some native users of /ɜ/ produce this stressed vowel with extended duration, that is, [ɜ :]. Alternatively, they may follow /ɜ/ with a brief /ə/ to create a diphthong, [ɜə]. For example, *person* could be produced as [pɜsən], [pɜ:sən], or [pɜəsən]. For the next exercise, transcribe the words with extended [ɜ:] and then with the [ɜə] diphthong. Pronounce each word after you transcribe it.

	[ɜ:]	[ɜə]
11. cursed	_____	_____
12. pearl	_____	_____
13. reserve	_____	_____
14. perch	_____	_____

	[ɜː]	[ɝə]
15. servant	_____	_____
16. curbs	_____	_____
17. German	_____	_____
18. absurd	_____	_____

Another feature of the dialect under consideration affects /ɹ/ following a vowel (postvocalic /ɹ/). In these words, the /ɹ/ will be omitted. (Note, however, that prevocalic and intervocalic /ɹ/ are produced in this dialect, just like mainstream American English. In words like *car* and *heart*, pronunciation would be [k ɑ] and [h ɑ t]. As with the /ɜ/ vowel sound, speakers may lengthen the vowel, for example, [k ɑ :], [hɑ: t], or add /ə/, for example, [k ɑ̄ə], [h ɑ̄ə t]. For the following words, transcribe them as they would be spoken by a person omitting postvocalic /ɹ/ sounds under each condition: omission, lengthening, /ə/ addition.

	[ ]	[ː]	[ə]
19. farm	_____	_____	_____
20. corn	_____	_____	_____
21. pairs	_____	_____	_____
22. sure	_____	_____	_____
23. there	_____	_____	_____
24. are	_____	_____	_____

One other dialectic variation is possible for postvocalic /ɹ/ when it follows a diphthong. In this case, /ə/ is commonly added in its place. Transcribe the following words with /ə/ substituted for /ɹ/.

25. hour _____		28. sour _____	
26. fire _____		29. spire _____	
27. choir _____		30. tower _____	

CHAPTER 20

REGIONAL DIALECTS
New England Dialect and /æ/ /ɑ/ /a/ /ɒ/

In New England and some other eastern dialects, the /ɑ/ is used in some words in which mainstream American English speakers would use /æ/. Consequently, *aunt* and *ask* would be pronounced as [ɑ n t] and [ɑ s k], respectively. Another vowel may also be used for such words, one that is made with a position between /æ/ and /ɑ/. Transcribed as /a/, it has the wide mouth opening of the /ɑ/ combined with elevation of the middle section of the tongue nearly as high as /æ/. It is used in Boston and in many parts of New England. If you are a mainstream American English speaker, you can produce /a/ by first placing your tongue in the position for /æ/. Then, open your mouth wider without changing tongue position. Or you can begin with the /ɑ/ position and raise the middle section of your tongue toward the /æ/ position. If you are able to produce the sound yourself, you can practice the exercises below on your own. If not, listen to a speaker who does make these distinctions in his or her speech.

A. PRODUCTION AND RECOGNITION

Pronounce (or listen to a practiced speaker pronounce) the following words aloud, observing the sequence indicated.

1. path   [p æ θ]   [p a θ]   [pɑ θ]
2. dance   [d ɑ nts] [d a nts] [d æ nts]
3. laugh   [l ɑ f]   [l æ f]   [l a f]
4. fast   [f æ st]   [f ɑ st]   [f a s t]
5. calf   [k a f]   [k ɑ f]   [k æ f]
6. can't   [k æ nt]   [k a nt]   [k ɑ n t]
7. ask   [ɑ s k]   [a s k]   [æ s k]
8. half   [h a f]   [h ɑ f]   [h ae f]

The /a/ is also commonly used in New England in place of /ɑ/ + postvocalic /r/ in words like *car* and *park*. Like the [ɑ :] in [k ɑ :], the /a/ may be extended, for example, [k a:], [p a: k]. If you are able to produce this sound, you can practice the exercises below yourself. If not, listen to a speaker who does make these distinctions in his or her speech.

9. park   [p ɑ r k]   [p a : k]   [p a k]   [p a : k]
10. barn   [b ɑ r n]   [b ɑ : n]   [b a n]   [b a : n]
11. jar   [ʤ ɑ r]   [ʤ ɑ :]   [ʤ a]   [ʤ a :]
12. Harvard [h ɑ r v ɚ d] [h ɑ : v ə d] [h a v əd]   [h a : v ə d]
13. market   [m ɑ r k ə t] [m ɑ : k ə t] [m a k ə t] [m a : k ə t]
14. tart   [t ɑ r t]   [t a : t]   [t a t]   [t a : t]

Another speech sound common to New England that is used in place of the mainstream /ɑ/ is the /ɒ/. The IPA symbol for this phoneme resembles a reversed and upside-down /ɑ/. Production for /ɒ/ is a shortened version of /ɑ/, but with slight lip rounding. It occurs most often in syllables spelled with *o* and ending in a stop consonant (e.g., *hot, stop*). It may also occur in words such as *watch, common, possible,* and *optimum.* If you do not typically use this phoneme, try beginning with the /ɑ/ position, and round your lips slightly (not as tensely as for /ɔ/) to produce /ɒ/. For the following exercise, you may produce the words aloud or listen to an experienced speaker produce them.

15. rot   [r ɑ t]   rot   [r ɒ t]   wrought [r ɔ t]
16. not   [n ɑ t]   not   [n ɒ t]   naught   [n ɔ t]
17. box   [b ɑ k s]   box   [b ɒ k s]   balks   [b ɔ k s]
18. nod   [n ɑ d]   nod   [n ɒ t]   gnawed   [n ɔ d]
19. popper [p ɑ pɚ]   popper [pɒ pə]   pauper   [p ɔ p ə]
20. cock   [k ɑ k]   cock   [k ɒ k]   caulk   [k ɔ k]

B. DISCRIMINATION

This exercise is designed to help you discriminate among the /ɑ/, /ɒ/, /a/, and other, more widely occurring American English vowels. Practice production of these lists (if you are able to produce all the vowels), or listen to a native user of [ɑr], [ɑ :], [a :], and [ɒ] produce them.

1. cart   [k ɑr t]   2. darn [d ɑr n]   3. hark [h ɑr k]
   cart   [k ɑ : t]   darn [d ɑ : n]   hark [h ɑ : k]
   cart   [k a : t]   darn [d a : n]   hark [h a : k]
   cat   [k æ t]   Dan   [d æ n]   hack [h æ k]
   coat   [k oʊ t]   down [d a ʊ n]   hook [h ʊ k]
   cot   [k ɑ t]   don   [d ɑ n]   hock [h ɑ k]
   cot   [k ɒ t]   don   [d ɒ n]   hock [h ɒ k]
   caught [k ɔ t]   dawn [d ɔ n]   hawk [h ɔ k]

INSTRUCTOR'S SECTION

CHAPTER 1: PREPARATORY LISTENING EXERCISES (pp. 5–7)

A. CONSONANT EXERCISES

1. (th)rew ma(sh) ba(th)e fu(dg)e ri(ch) ha(ng)
   bru(sh) (ph)one mo(th) si(ng)s bo(th) th(is)
2. pe(pp)er se(ss)ion se(tt)ing mu(tt) ca(rr)y
   fa(ll)ing hu(gg)ed be(ll) sli(pp)ed mu(ff)
3. com(b) (k)nife (p)neumonia (p)sychology (g)nome
   (g)nat (p)salm paradi(g)m autum(n)
4. a. chorus chic b. lose pose c. gang buggy
5. a. zebra   tons   whose   busy   /z/
   b. machine   ocean   shelf   issue   /ʃ/
   c. engine   joy   fudge   giant   /ʤ/
   d. tax   scissors racer   person   /s/
   e. young   few   William   onion   /j/
   f. who   high   ahead   whole   /h/
   g. trough   full   phone   graph   /f/
   h. anger   grow   lager   pig   /g/

B. VOWEL EXERCISES

1. r(oa)d (ou)tside s(ou)py p(ai)d c(oa)ster m(ou)nded
   br(oo)d c(oi)led r(ai)ning vacat(io)n racc(oo)n b(oa)ting
2. cod(e) rag(e)d foster(e)d troup(e) etch(e)d fum(e)
3. a. yellow b. shoe c. bear
4. a. rain   skein   pane   patriot   /eɪ/
   b. police   secret   peanuts   beetle   /i/
   c. wrap   sat   banana   ashes   /æ/
   d. hoop   grew   moose   flume   /u/
   e. possum   pap   bond   soggy   /ɑ/
   f. nut   ton   under   double   /ʌ/
   g. bitter   rich   indigo   picture   /ɪ/
   h. wood   could   took   full   /ʊ/

5. a. 5   b.   3   c. f/i/n/d 4   d. s/u/mm/er/ 4   e. i/n/k/ 3
   f. k/i/te/ 3   g. e/gg/ 2   h. s/p/ee/ch/ 4
   i. b/o/k/s 3   j. c/ur/ve/ 3   k. t/a/pe/ 3   l. s/u/n/ 3
6. a. choke → coach   b. tube → boot   c. chirp → perch
   d. keys → Zeke   e. lash → shall   f. zoo → ooze
   g. cub → buck   h. I'd → die   i. scat → tacks

CHAPTER 2: TRANSCRIPTION OF FRONT VOWELS (pp. 11–13)

A. RECOGNITION

List 1: /ɪ/   List 2: /æ/   List 3: /i/   List 4: /ɛ/   List 5: /i/   List 6: /ɪ/

B. DISCRIMINATION

List 1 /i/:   eve   tea   chief   marine   demon
List 2 /ɪ/:   myth   kitchen   business   itched   gym   bitter   sieve   lift
List 3 /e/:   Kool-Aid   indicate   alligator   renovate   landscape
List 4 /ɛ/:   hen   red   belt   friend   many   men
List 5 /æ/:   can   apple   knack   half   backed   camera

C. WORD TRANSCRIPTION FROM SPELLING/DICTATION

EXERCISE 1: FRONT VOWEL CONTRAST DRILLS

List A: /i/–/ɪ/	List B: /i/–/ɛ/	List C: /ɪ/–/ɛ/
1. [i] [ɪ]	1. [i] [ɛ]	1. [ɪ] [ɛ]
2. [i] [ɪ]	2. [ɛ] [i]	2. [ɛ] [ɪ]
3. [ɪ] [i]	3. [ɛ] [i]	3. [ɪ] [ɛ]
4. [ɪ] [i]	4. [ɛ] [i]	4. [ɛ] [ɪ]
5. [i] [ɪ]	5. [i] [ɛ]	5. [ɪ] [ɛ]
6. [i] [ɪ]	6. [ɛ] [i]	6. [ɛ] [ɪ]
7. [i] [ɪ]	7. [i] [ɛ]	7. [ɛ] [ɪ]
8. [ɪ] [i]	8. [i] [ɛ]	8. [ɪ] [ɛ]

List D: /ɛ/–/æ/	List E: /æ/–/ɑ/
1. [ɛ] [æ]	1. [æ] [ɑ]
2. [ɛ] [æ]	2. [æ] [ɑ]
3. [æ] [ɛ]	3. [ɑ] [æ]
4. [ɛ] [æ]	4. [ɑ] [æ]
5. [ɛ] [æ]	5. [æ] [ɑ]
6. [ɛ] [æ]	6. [ɑ] [æ]
7. [æ] [ɛ]	7. [ɑ] [æ]
8. [æ] [ɛ]	8. [æ] [ɑ]

EXERCISE 2: FRONT VOWELS

1. [ɪ]	9. [ɛ]	17. [i]	25. [ɪ]
2. [æ]	10. [ɪ]	18. [æ]	26. [ɛ]
3. [ɛ]	11. [æ]	19. [ɪ]	27. [i]
4. [i]	12. [æ]	20. [ɛ]	28. [æ]
5. [ɛ]	13. [i]	21. [i]	29. [ɛ]
6. [ɪ]	14. [ɪ]	22. [ɪ]	30. [i]
7. [æ]	15. [ɛ]	23. [æ]	
8. [i]	16. [ɪ]	24. [ɛ]	

D. WORD TRANSCRIPTION FROM LIVE DICTATION

1.	scene	[ɪ]	11.	gripping	[ɪ ɪ]
2.	intent	[ɪ ɛ]	12.	thick	[ɪ]
3.	enchanting	[ɛ æ ɪ]	13.	fascist	[æ ɪ]
4.	invents	[ɪ ɛ]	14.	plenty	[ɛ i]
5.	whims	[ɪ]	15.	switching	[ɪ ɪ]
6.	these	[i]	16.	bag	[æ]
7.	many	[ɛ i]	17.	prestige	[ɛ i]
8.	rapid	[æ ɪ]	18.	cab	[æ]
9.	pity	[ɪ i]	19.	bewitched	[i ɪ]
10.	last	[æ]	20.	yeast	[i]

CHAPTER 3: TRANSCRIPTION OF BACK VOWELS (pp. 15–17)

A. RECOGNITION

List 1: /ʊ/   List 2: /ɑ/   List 3: /o/   List 4: /u/   List 5: /ɔ/

B. DISCRIMINATION

List 1 /u/: tomb chewed cruiser blue doom soup cute
List 2 /ʊ/: wool pull hooked put good full
List 3 /ɔ/: naught pawnshop call hawk bawl ball caught
List 4 /ɑ/: common honor alms psalm father sob oddity

C. WORD TRANSCRIPTION FROM SPELLING/DICTATION

EXERCISE 1: BACK VOWEL CONTRAST DRILLS

List A: /u/–/ʊ/	List B: /ɔ/–/ɑ/	List C: /ɑ/–/æ/
1. [ʊ] [u]	1. [ɑ] [ɔ]	1. [ɑ] [æ]
2. [u] [ʊ]	2. [ɔ] [ɑ]	2. [æ] [ɑ]
3. [u] [ʊ]	3. [ɔ] [ɑ]	3. [æ] [ɑ]
4. [ʊ] [u]	4. [ɔ] [ɑ]	4. [ɑ] [æ]
5. [ʊ] [u]	5. [ɑ] [ɔ]	5. [æ] [ɑ]
6. [u] [ʊ]	6. [ɑ] [ɔ]	6. [ɑ] [æ]
7. [u] [ʊ]	7. [ɔ] [ɑ]	7. [æ] [ɑ]
8. [ʊ] [u]	8. [ɑ] [ɔ]	8. [æ] [ɑ]

EXERCISE 2: FRONT AND BACK VOWELS

1. [u]	11. [ɛ ɑ]	21. [ʊ]
2. [ʊ ɛ]	12. [ɑ]	22. [u i]
3. [ɔ ʊ]	13. [æ ɔ]	23. [ɔ]
4. [ɑ ɪ]	14. [ʊ ɪ]	24. [æ ʊ]
5. [ɑ ɪ]	15. [ɑ]	25. [u]
6. [ɔ i]	16. [ʊ]	26. [u]
7. [æ u]	17. [u]	27. [ɔ]
8. [ɔ]	18. [i ɔ]	28. [ʊ]
9. [ɑ i]	19. [ɔ ɪ]	29. [ɑ]
10. [ʊ]	20. [u]	30. [ɑ i]

D. WORD TRANSCRIPTION FROM LIVE DICTATION

1. thaw [ɔ]	6. wood [ʊ]	11. gone [ɔ]	16. knocked [ɑ]
2. should [ʊ]	7. bomb [ɑ]	12. prawns [ɔ]	17. rouge [u]
3. whom [u]	8. olive [ɑ ɪ]	13. ostrich [ɑ ɪ]	18. tune [u]
4. yawn [ɔ]	9. choose [u]	14. knocking [ɑ ɪ]	19. beautiful [u ɪ ʊ]
5. vault [ɔ]	10. absolving [æ ɑ ɪ]	15. smooth [u]	20. goods [ʊ]

CHAPTER 4: TRANSCRIPTION OF CENTRAL VOWELS (pp. 18–20)

A. RECOGNITION

List 1: /ɝ/   List 2: /ʌ/   List 3: /ɚ/   List 4: /ə/

B. DISCRIMINATION

List 1 /ʌ/:   dull   ugly   mother   come   son   does
List 2 /ə/:   diction   awesome   banana   tunnel   again   lemon   attuned
List 3 /ɝ/:   fur   word   turned   thorough   curried   girl   dessert
List 4 /ɚ/:   supper   tailor   pusher   zither   manner   nearer

C. WORD TRANSCRIPTION FROM SPELLING/DICTATION

EXERCISE 1: CENTRAL VOWEL COMPARISON DRILLS

List A: /ɝ/–/ɚ/   List B: /ʌ/–/ə/

1. [u ɚ]	1. [ʌ ə]
2. [ɝ e]	2. [ʌ ə]
3. [ɝ i]	3. [ə u ɪ ə]
4. [ɝ]	4. [ʌ i]
5. [ɔ ɚ]	5. [ʌ u]
6. [ɝ]	6. [ə ɑ ɪ]
7. [ɝ ɚ]	7. [ə i]
8. [ɝ ɚ i]	8. [ʌ i]
9. [æ ɚ]	9. [i ə]
10. [i ɪ ɚ]	10. [ə u]

EXERCISE 2: FRONT, BACK, AND CENTRAL VOWELS

1. [æ ɪ ʌ ɚ]   11. [ɝ u]   21. [æ ɚ]
2. [i i ɚ]   12. [i ɝ]   22. [ə ɛ]
3. [ɝ ɪ]   13. [ə oʊ ɚ]   23. [ʌ æ]
4. [ʌ ɚ]   14. [ɝ ə]   24. [ʌ]
5. [ɛ ə ɑ ɚ]   15. [ə u ɚ]   25. [i ʌ]
6. [ɝ ɪ]   16. [ʌ ɚ]   26. [ʌ]
7. [ɝ ə]   17. [ɝ]   27. [ɝ i]
8. [ʌ ɚ]   18. [ʌ]   28. [ɝ ɪ]
9. [ʌ ɚ]   19. [ʌ ɑ]   29. [ɝ i]
10. [æ ɚ ɚ]   20. [ʌ ɚ ə]   30. [i ɚ]

D. WORD TRANSCRIPTION FROM LIVE DICTATION: FRONT, BACK, AND CENTRAL VOWELS

1. shoved [ʌ]   6. month [ʌ]   11. bother [ɑ ɚ]   16. mustard [ʌ ɚ]
2. faster [æ ɚ]   7. avert [ə ɝ]   12. leisure [i ɚ]   17. salmon [æ ə]
3. pleasure [ɛ ɚ]   8. attorney [ə ɝ i] 13. lurk [ɝ]   18. again [ə ɛ]
4. early [ɝ i]   9. younger [ʌ ɚ]   14. running [ʌ ɪ]   19. oven [ʌ ə]
5. justice [ʌ ə]   10. booster [u ɚ] 15. wonder [ʌ ɚ]   20. learner [ɝ ɚ]

CHAPTER 5: VOWELS AND DIPHTHONGS (pp. 21–23)

A. RECOGNITION

1. Rising Diphthongs

List A: /eɪ/   List B: /oʊ/   List C: /aʊ/   List D: /ɔɪ/   List E: /aɪ/

2. Centering Diphthongs

List A: /ɑɚ/   List B: /ɪɚ/   List C: /ʊɚ/   List D: /ɔɚ   List E: /ɛɚ/

B. DISCRIMINATION

1. Rising Diphthongs

List A: /eɪ/: danger   prey   eighty   katydid   payment   matinee
List B: /oʊ/: hoping   donut   loner   coast   thrown
List C: /aʊ/: count   foundry   powder   bower   pouch
List D: /ɔɪ/: poise   hoist   boyish   avoidance
List E: /aɪ/: highly   kindness   binder   minded   rhinoceros   child

2. Centering Diphthongs

List A: /ɔɚ/: courtship   boarded   hoarse   border   torch
List B: /ɪɚ/: fear   dear   sheer   near   gear   hearing
List C: /ʊɚ/: bear   airplane   careful   rare   stairs
List D: /ɑɚ/: hardest   partner   Farsi   gardener   parsnip   heartened
               marvelous

C. Word Transcription from Spelling/Dictation: All Vowels and Rising Diphthongs

1. [aɪ]	11. [eɪ]	21. [aʊ ɪ]
2. [eɪ]	12. [ɔɪ]	22. [aɪ ɛ]
3. [ɔɪ]	13. [ɔɪ]	23. [ɔɪ]
4. [aɪ]	14. [eɪ]	24. [i aʊ]
5. [aʊ i]	15. [oʊ i]	25. [ə eɪ]
6. [ɔɪ ə i]	16. [aɪ ə]	26. [aɪ i]
7. [aʊ]	17. [aʊ]	27. [aʊ ɪ]
8. [eɪ ɪ]	18. [oʊ ə]	28. [ə oʊ]
9. [ʌ aʊ]	19. [aɪ ɚ]	29. [i aɪ]
10. [ə aɪ]	20. [eɪ]	30. [aʊ ɚ]

D. Word Transcription from Live Dictation

1.	voices	[ɔɪ ə]	11.	white	[aɪ]
2.	opener	[oʊ ə ɚ]	12.	Thursday	[ɝ eɪ]
3.	mindful	[aɪ ʊ]	13.	beige	[eɪ]
4.	hounding	[aʊ ɪ]	14.	chime	[aɪ]
5.	stray	[eɪ]	15.	coil	[ɔɪ]
6.	rejoice	[i ɔɪ]	16.	yolk	[oʊ]
7.	loiter	[ɔɪ ɚ]	17.	today	[u eɪ]
8.	those	[oʊ]	18.	grouse	[aʊ]
9.	game	[eɪ]	19.	nightfall	[aɪ]
10.	crowd	[aʊ]	20.	exploit	[ɛ ɔɪ]

CHAPTER 6: TRANSCRIPTION OF STOP CONSONANTS (pp. 27–29)

A. Recognition

List 1: /k/   List 2: /d/   List 3: /t/   List 4: /b/   List 5: /g/   List 6: /p/

B. Discrimination

List 1: /p/:   apple   spring   hopped   paper   upon
List 2: /b/:   rabbit   mob   absolved   bomb   bright   ebony
List 3: /t/:   doubt   Thomas   laughed   liked   ptomaine   antler
List 4: /d/:   adore   medal   Wednesday   should   middle   bathed
List 5: /k/:   baroque   accord   chasm   accident   taxi   liquid
List 6: /g/:   again   finger   ghost   example   bragged   rogue

C. Word Transcription from Spelling/Dictation: Stops, Vowels, Diphthongs

1. [p eɪ d]	7. [g ʌ]
2. [b ʌ g i]	8. [g æ d ɑ]
3. [k ʌ b]	9. [t oʊd]
4. [g ɑ d]	10. [t i p ɑ t]
5. [k æ ʊ]	11. [d ɪ p t]
6. [g ʊ d i]	12. [k aɪ t]

13. [k oʊ p eɪ]   22. [b ə t ɑ]
14. [g æ b]   23. [p ɪ t]
15. [b æ d]   24. [k ɑ p i]
16. [b ɪ g ə t]   25. [g ɛ t]
17. [p ɔ d]   26. [g æ p]
18. [d ɝ t]   27. [g oʊ d]
19. [b ɔ t]   28. [b aɪ k ɚ]
20. [b æ d æ ə]   29. [k ʌ p k eɪ k]
21. [k ʌ t ɚ]   30. [d ɛ k e d]

D. Word Transcription from Live Dictation

1. pod	[p ɑ d]	11. chemist	[k ɛ m ɪ t][1]
2. bag	[b æ g]	12. technique	[t ɛ k i k]
3. taped	[t eɪ p t]	13. cupboard	[k ʌ b ɚ d]
4. Quaker	[k eɪ k ɚ]	14. steep	[t i p]
5. gap	[g æ p]	15. biggest	[b ɪ g ɛ t][1]
6. curb	[k ɝ b]	16. abdicate	[æ b d ɪ k eɪ t][1]
7. wiggle	[ɪ g ʊ]	17. puppet	[p ʌ p ə t]
8. clipped	[k ɪ p t]	18. cargo	[k ɑ g o ʊ]
9. gable	[g eɪ b ʊ]	19. downtown	[d aʊ t aʊ]
10. adapt	[ə d æ p t]	20. madrigal	[æ d ɪ gʊ]

CHAPTER 7: FRICATIVES (pp. 30–33)

1. Exercises for Fricative Cognate Pairs: /f/–/v/ /θ/–/ð/ and /h/

A. Recognition

List 1: /ð/   List 2: /f/   List 3: /v/   List 4: /θ/   List 5: /h/

B. Discrimination

List 1 /f/: coffee elephant fifteen prophet half fault infant farm
List 2 /v/: valet vacuum driver halves divide of vase
List 3 /θ/: booth thigh anthem south thorny myth
List 4 /ð/: these they'll weather bathe clothes[2] heathen bathe
List 5 /h/: who behind half hope behave Ohio

C. Word Transcription from Spelling/Dictation:
/f/–/v/   /θ/–/ð/   /h/

1. [f ʊ t]   7. [b r i ð]
2. [i l ɛ v ə θ] 8. [f ɔ θ]
3. [h oʊ p f ʊ l] 9. [f eɪ t]
4. [t i θ]   10. [h i ð ə]
5. [v ɪ v ɪ d][3] 11. [b ɝ θ d eɪ]
6. [f ɑðɚ h ʊ d] 12. [b i v ɚ]

---

[1]Second vowel may be produced as [ə].
[2]Inclusion of /ð/ depends on dialect.
[3]Second vowel may be produced as /ə/.

13. [p æ θ eɪ]   17. [θ ɝ t i]
14. [f ɔ θ]   18. [h ʌ f]
15. [v ɪ k t ɚ]   19. [f eɪ θ]
16. [b ɑ ð ɚ]   20. [ð eɪ v]

2. EXERCISES FOR FRICATIVE COGNATE PAIRS: /s/–/z/   /ʃ/–/ʒ/

A. RECOGNITION

List 1: /ʒ/   List 2: /z/   List 3: /s/   List 4: /ʃ/

B. DISCRIMINATION

List 1: /s/:   racer   mouse   icing   escape   precious   feast   loose
List 2: /z/:   enzyme   misery   zigzag   rose   visible   fused   clothes
List 3: /ʃ/:   insurance   pressure   caution   washed   tissue   fresh
List 4: /ʒ/:   treasure   confusion   beige   leisure   usual   casual

C. WORD TRANSCRIPTION FROM SPELLING/DICTATION: /s/–/z/   /ʃ/–/ʒ/

1. [s æ ʃ]   8. [p ɛ ʃ ɚ]   15. [ɪ ʃ]
2. [z u k i p ɚ]   9. [p ɛʒ ɚ]   16. [oʊz oʊ]
3. [m ɛ ʒ ɚ d]   10. [v ɪ ʃ ə s]   17. [i z i ɚ]
4. [s i ʃ ɛ]   11. [p ɛ ʃ ə s]   18. [s i ʒ ɚ]
5. [æ ʒ ɚ]   12. [p i t z ə]   19. [g eɪ z d]
6. [ʃ i t s]   13. [t ɛʒ ɚ d]   20. [s ɪ s t ɚ]
7. [ʃ u z]   14. [p ɝ ʒ ə]

D. WORD TRANSCRIPTION FROM LIVE DICTATION: FRICATIVES, STOPS, VOWELS, AND DIPHTHONGS

1. fastest   [fæ s t ɪ s t][1]   11. brotherhood   [b ʌ ð ɚ h ʊ d]
2. vacation   [v e k eɪ ʃ ə]   12. confusion   [k ə f u ʒ ə n]
3. toothbrush   [t u θ b ʌ ʃ]   13. husband   [h ʌ z b ə d]
4. hover   [h ʌ v ɚ]   14. garage   [g ə ɑ ʒ]
5. corsage   [k ɔ s ɑ ʒ]   15. shoelace   [ʃ u e s]
6. themselves   [ð ɛ s ɛ v z]   16. frothy   [f ɔ θi]
7. shift   [ʃ ɪ f t]   17. phonate   [f oʊ e t]
8. aspersion   [æ s p ɝ ʒ ə n]   18. mustache   [ʌ s t æ ʃ]
9. birthplace   [b ɝ θ p eɪ s]   19. explosion   [ɛ k s p oʊ ʒ ə]
10. father   [f ɑ ð ɚ]   20. Thursday   [θ ɝ z d eɪ]

CHAPTER 8: AFFRICATES: /tʃ/ /dʒ/ (pp. 34–35)

A. RECOGNITION

List 1: /dʒ/   List 2: /tʃ/   List 3: /tʃ/   List 4: /dʒ/

---

[1]/ə/ may replace second vowel, depending on dialectic variation.

B. Discrimination

List 1: /ʧ/: scratch natural cheap capture lecture kitchen catcher
List 2: /ʤ/: large angel bungee jealous enjoy larger
List 3: /ʧ/: chipmunk teacher chain charge pitch patch
List 4: /ʤ/: jealous injure zoology ranger graduate engine

C. Word Transcription from Spelling/Dictation: Affricates, Fricatives, Stops, Vowels, and Diphthongs

1. [s t ɪ ʧ ɛ z][1]
2. [d ɑ ʤ]
3. [ʧ aɪ d h ʊ d]
4. [ʧ ɑ p s t ɪ k s]
5. [t ʌ ʤ i]
6. [s ʌ b ʤ ɛ k t]
7. [a ʤ ɚ]
8. [ʧ aɪ v z]
9. [oʊ v ɚ ʧ ɚ]
10. [ʤ eɪ k ə b]
11. [p æ ʧ ɚ k]
12. [b æ d ɪ ʤ][1]
13. [æ d v ɛ ʧ ɚ]
14. [s p i ʧ]
15. [θ i ɑ ə ʤ i]
16. [b æ ʤ]
17. [s k æ ʧ t]
18. [ʧ i k]
19. [ʤ ɚ k t]
20. [t æ ʤ ɚ i][2]
21. [ʧ eɪ s t]
22. [f ɛ ʧ f aɪ z]
23. [ʧ i z k eɪ k]
24. [k æ b ɪ ʤ][1]
25. [s t ɛ ʧ t]
26. [g ʌ ʤ]
27. [v ɛ ʧ ɚ d]
28. [p æ s ɛ ʤ ɚ][1]
29. [ʧ æ ɪ ʤ][1]
30. [ʧ eɪ ʤ]

D. Word Transcription from Live Dictation

1.	hitch	[h ɪ ʧ]	11.	gauge	[g eɪ ʤ]
2.	adjust	[æ ʤ ʌ s t]	12.	jeans	[ʤ i z]
3.	village	[v ɪ ɪ ʤ][1]	13.	thatched	[θ æ ʧ t]
4.	barged	[b ɑ ʤ d]	14.	China	[ʧ aɪ ə]
5.	image	[ɪ ɪ ʤ][1]	15.	recheck	[i ʧ ɛ k]
6.	catcher	[k æ ʧ ɚ]	16.	pajamas	[p ə ʤ æ ə z][3]
7.	jade	[ʤ eɪ d]	17.	scourge	[s k ɚ ʤ]
8.	future	[f u ʧ ɚ]	18.	fractured	[f æ k ʧ ɚ d]
9.	chews	[ʧ u z]	19.	gotcha	[g ɑʧ ə]
10.	checkbook	[ʧ ɛ k b ʊ k]	20.	nudge	[ʌ ʤ]

CHAPTER 9: NASALS: /m/ /n/ /ŋ/ (pp. 36–38)

A. Recognition

List 1: /n/   List 2: /ŋ/   List 3: /m/

---

[1]Second vowel may be produced as /ə/, depending on dialect.
[2]May also be produced as [t æ ʤ ə i] (*tangerine*).
[3]Second vowel may be produced as /ɑ/, depending on dialect.

B. DISCRIMINATION

List 1: /m/: calm infamous diaphragm summer pneumonia prism mnemonic
numb
List 2: /n/: knob gnash reign gnat cringe
List 3: /ŋ/: anxious angle donkey think song single singing

C. WORD TRANSCRIPTION FROM SPELLING/DICTATION: NASALS, AFFRICATES, FRICATIVES, STOPS, VOWELS, AND DIPHTHONGS

1. [m i t ɚ]	16. [h ɪ m s ɛ f]
2. [g æ ŋ]	17. [ɛ v i θ ɪ ŋ]
3. [k oʊ m ɪ ŋ]	18. [s ʌ m t aɪ m z]
4. [r i m u v]	19. [k æ n t ɚ]
5. [tʃ ɪ m ni]	20. [s ɪ ŋ ʃ ɑ t]
6. [m ɛ n t]	21. [s t ʌ n ɪ ŋ]
7. [ɪ n f i d]	22. [n eɪ ʃ ə n]
8. [t eɪ k ɪ ŋ]	23. [ə m ɛ n d]
9. [s ɪ ŋ ɚ]	24. [n u m æ t ɪ k]¹
10. [ʌ n z]	25. [s m u ð]
11. [d ɑ m ə]	26. [ð ɛ n]
12. [k ə m p i t]	27. [ɔ ŋ g ɚ]
13. [s æ n d ɪ ŋ]	28. [h ɛ d ɪ ŋ]
14. [s m oʊ k ɪ ŋ]	29. [m oʊ t ɚ]
15. [h æ ŋ ɚ z]	30. [m i n ɪ ŋ f ʊ]

D. WORD TRANSCRIPTION FROM LIVE DICTATION

1.	patching	[p æ tʃ ɪ ŋ]	11.	judging	[dʒ ʌ dʒ ɪ ŋ]
2.	manner	[m æ n ɚ]	12.	bonanza	[b ə n æ n z ə]³
3.	breathing	[b r i ð ɪ ŋ]	13.	memories	[m ɛ m ɚ i z]
4.	human	[h u m ə n]	14.	Minnesota	[m ɪ n ə s oʊ t ə]
5.	thickening	[θ ɪ k ɛ n ɪ ŋ]²	15.	English	[ɪ ŋ g ɪ ʃ]
6.	monster	[m ɑ n s t ɚ]	16.	Band-Aid	[b æ n d eɪ d]
7.	venom	[v ɛ n ə m]	17.	tongue	[t ʌ ŋ]
8.	minimizing	[m ɪ n ɪ m aɪ z ɪ ŋ]²	18.	domain	[d o m eɪ n]
9.	cranky	[k r æ ŋ k i]	19.	grandma	[g æ n d m ə]
10.	sound	[s aʊ n d]	20.	mining	[m aɪ n ɪ ŋ]

CHAPTER 10: ORAL RESONANT CONSONANTS: GLIDES AND LIQUIDS (pp. 39–42)

A. RECOGNITION

List 1: /l/   List 2: /j/   List 3: /w/   List 4: /r/

---

¹[ə] may replace [ɪ].
²Second vowel may be [ə] in some dialects.
³[o] may replace [ə] in first syllable.

B. Discrimination

1. Liquids and Glides

List A /w/: reward memoirs anywhere[1] linguist William watt dwell
List B /j/: youthful canyon union beauty few yeast pewter view
List C /l/: gale gulp tulip teller lilac twelve wall dearly
List D /r/: rhyme try carrot bread crowded rhythm Barry treasure

2. Consonant /r/ versus /ɚ/-Diphthongs

a. Postvocalic /r/

1.	car	[k ɑ r]	[k ɑ ɚ]
2.	bear	[b ɛ r]	[b ɛɚ]
3.	torn	[t ɔ r n]	[t ɔɚ n]
4.	fierce	[f ɪ r s]	[f ɪɚ s]
5.	party	[p ɑ r t i]	[p ɑɚ t i]
6.	yearly	[j ɪ r l i]	[j ɪɚ l i]
7.	morning	[m ɔ r n ɪ ŋ]	[m ɔɚ n.ɪ ŋ]
8.	partake	[p ɑ r t eɪ k]	[p ɑɚ t eɪ k]
9.	dared	[d ɛ r d]	[d ɛɚ d]
10.	cheer	[tʃ ɪ r]	[tʃ ɪɚ]

b. Vowels /ɝ/ /ɚ/ and Consonantal /r/

List 1 /r/: range gray arrow prayer trailer cream frog
List 2 /ɚ/: hammer dryer understand preacher overcoat
List 3 /ɝ/: birch turn murder return burn wordy
List 4 /r/: trustee broken tearing processor afraid crowd regal

c. Consonant /r/ and Vowels /ɝ/ /ɚ/

1. [k ɝ t ə n]   6. [f ɝ n ə s]
   [kɑr t ə n]   [f ɛ r n ə s]
2. [h ɝ i]   7. [f ɝ m ɪ ŋ]
   [h ɛ r i]   [f ɑ r m ɪ ŋ]
3. [k ɛ r ʊ l]   8. [p ɑ r k]
   [k ɝ l]   [p ɝ k]
4. [f ɝ i]   9. [k ɝ b]
   [f ɛ r i]   [k ɛ r ə b]
5. [h ɑ r t s] 10. [w ɝ m]
   [h ɝ t s]   [w ɔ r m]

---

[1][ʍ] rather than [w] may be used.

C. Word Transcription from Spelling/Dictation: All Consonants, Vowels, and Diphthongs

1. [l ɑ ʤ ɪ ŋ]
2. [w ɪ ʧ]
3. [r eɪ d ɑ r]
4. [l aɪ l æ k]
5. [j i l d]
6. [f r ɔ g]
7. [f r i w eɪ]
8. [w ɑ t ɚ]
/9. [r ɛ l ə t ɪ v]
10. [w ɪ ʃ ɪ ŋ]
11. [t aʊ w ʊ l]
12. [p r aʊ d]
13. [f j u ʧ ɚ]
14. [d w ɪ n d ʊ l]
15. [r ɔɪ j ʊ l]
16. [w i k l i]
17. [k j u t]
18. [l æ f]
19. [v æ l j ə b ʊ l]
20. [l æ k ɪ ŋ]
21. [j u θ f ʊ l]
22. [j e l oʊ]
23. [k j u b ɪ k]
24. [j ɑ r n]
25. [j u s f ʊ l]
26. [k ɑ l ɚ]
27. [w ɪ n t ɚ]
28. [s æ n d w ɪ ʧ]
29. [w oʊ v ə n]
30. [r i æ k t]

D. Word Transcription from Live Dictation

1. cued   [k j u d]
2. relation   [r i l eɪ ʃ ə n]
3. millions   [m ɪ l j ə n z]
4. wealthy   [w ɛ l θ i]
5. unused   [ə n j u z d]
6. clothing   [k l oʊ ð ɪ ŋ]
7. farm   [f ɑ r m]
8. restless   [r ɛ s t l ɛ s][1]
9. William   [w ɪ l j ə m]
10. grapes   [g r eɪ p s]
11. truly   [t r u l i]
12. rolling   [r oʊ l ɪ ŋ]
13. cloth   [k l ɔ θ]
14. fugitive   [f j u ʤ ɪ t ɪ v][1]
15. rather   [r æ ð ɚ]
16. likely   [l aɪ k l i]
17. fertilizer   [f ɝ t ɪ l aɪ z ɚ][1]
18. wagered   [w eɪ ʤ ɚ d]
19. flavor   [f l eɪ v ɚ]
20. wheel   [w i l][2]

CHAPTER 11: ALTERATIONS IN DURATION (pp. 45–46)

A. Narrow Transcription: Lengthening in Phrases

1. [b oʊ θ : ʌ m z]
2. [b ɑ r : eɪ]
3. [h æ f : ʊ l]
4. [s ʌ m : aɪ s]
5. [k ɔ l : ɪ n d ə]
6. [t w ɛ v : aʊ l z]
7. [b æ n : u k s]
8. [s eɪ m : ɛ n]
9. [b eɪ ð : ɛ m]
10. [h ɪ z : ɪ p ɚ z]

---

[1]Second vowel may be [ə].

[2][ʍ] may replace [w].

B. Narrow Transcription: Syllabic Consonants

1. [k æ t ʊ l]   [k æ t l̩]
2. [m ɪ t n̩]   [m ɪ t ə n]
3. [h ʌ d l̩]   [h ʌ d ʊ l]
4. [f r oʊ z ə n]   [f r oʊ z n̩]
5. [b ʌ t ə n]   [b ʌ t n̩]
6. [s ɔ f ə n]   [s ɔ f n̩]
7. [b ɑ t ə l]   [b ɑ t l̩]
8. [h æ s l̩]   [h æ s ʊ l]
9. [t ɑ p l̩]   [t ɑ p ʊ l]
10. [k eɪ b ʊ l]   [k eɪ b l̩]
11. [l eɪ d l̩]   [l eɪ d ʊ l]
12. [s n ɪ f l̩]   [s n ɪ f ʊ l]
13. [s ɪ m p l̩]   [s ɪ m p ʊ l]
14. [s æ t ɪ n]   [s æ t n̩]
15. [k ɑ t n̩]   [k ɑ t ə n]

CHAPTER 12: ASPIRATION OF STOPS (pp. 47–49)

A. Narrow Transcription of Singleton Stops

1. [pʰ ɑ p˺]   [pʰ ɑ pʰ]
2. [tʰ ɑɪ pʰ]   [tʰ ɑɪ p˺]
3. [h æ t˺]   [h æ tʰ]
4. [s i tʰ]   [s i t˺]
5. [pʰ i k˺]   [pʰ i kʰ]
6. [l u p˺]   [l u pʰ]
7. [f ɔ t˺]   [f ɔ tʰ]
8. [b eɪ tʰ]   [b eɪ t˺]
9. [kʰ ɑ t˺]   [kʰ ɑ tʰ]
10. [kʰ oʊ pʰ]   [kʰ oʊ p˺]
11. [s oʊ pʰ]   [s oʊ p˺]
12. [ʃ ɑ k˺]   [ʃ ɑ kʰ]
13. [s ɛ tʰ]   [s ɛ t˺]
14. [r oʊ t˺]   [r oʊ tʰ]

B. Narrow Transcription of Stop Sequences

1. [kʰ ɛ p˺ tʰ]   11. [h ɑ t˺ːʰ ʌ b]
2. [h ɑ t˺ kʰ ɑ r]   12. [ð æ t˺ kʰ ɑ r]
3. l æ p˺ tʰ ɑ p˺]   13. [ɪ n tʰ u]
4. [d ɔ n tʰ]   14. [s ɪp˺ tʰ]
5. l æ k˺ tʰ]   15. [kʰ æ n tʰ]
6. [l ɪ m pʰ]   16. [ð æ t˺ pʰ ɛ r]
7. [s æ ŋ kʰ]   17. [kʰ ɪ k˺ tʰ]
8. [pʰ eɪ s tʰ]   18. [kʰ æ m pʰ]
9. [pʰ ɑɪ n kʰ oʊ n]   19. [w ɑ s pʰ]
10. [l i k˺ tʰ]   20. [m ɪ s tʰ]

C. Narrow Transcription of Stops: Singletons and Sequences

1. [eɪ kʰɔ r n]
2. [kʰeɪ k ʰ]
3. [b æ kˀ pʰ ɔ r ʧ]
4. [h ɑ pʰ ɪ ŋ]
5. [pʰ eɪ m ə n tʰ]
6. [kʰ oʊ tˀ :ʰ eɪ l z]
7. [s pˀ ɝ tʰ]
8. [s tˀ ʌ k ʰɪ]
9. [l æ s tʰ]
10. [pʰɑ pˀ t ʰɑpˀ]

11. [æ p ʰ l̩]
12. [s kˀ ɪ pˀ]
13. [r i kʰ ʌ v ɚ]
14. [pʰ ɑpˀkʰɔr n]
15. [kʰ ʌ s pʰ]
16. [r ɛ n tʰ]
17. [tʰ eɪ kˀ :ʰ ɛ r]
18. [ʃ ɔ r tʰ]
19. [l æ f tʰ]
20. [pʰʌ pʰi]

CHAPTER 13: ASSIMILATORY CHANGES: PLACE AND RESONANCE (pp. 50–51)

A. Dentalization

1. [wʌ n̪ θʌm]
2. [b oʊ θ t̪ aɪ z]
3. [k oʊ d̪ð ɛ m]
4. [eɪ t̪ θ s̪ t a r]
5. [w ɪ θ t̪ ɑm]
6. [m ɔ θ t̪ r æ p]
7. [b æ θ s̪ oʊ p]
8. [r aɪ d̪ð ɛ r]

9. [ɪ n̪ ð ɛ r]
10. [k l̩ ɔ θ t̪ aʊ w ʊ l]
11. [l u z̪ð ɛ m]
12. [s aʊ θ t̪ oʊ l]
13. [a n̪ ð ɪ s]
14. [i v ə n̪ ð oʊ]
15. [f ɔ r θ t̪ aɪ m]
16. [h ɛ l̩ θ t̪ɛ k s t]

B. Other Assimilatory Place Shifts

1. [p l eɪ ʃ :ɪf t]
2. [m ɪ ʃ : i l ə]
3. [p æ ʧ: ɔ k]
4. [m aʊ ʃ ʧ i z]
5. [b ɛ n ʧ ʃ t r i t]

6. [f ʌ ʤ ʃ ʌ n d eɪ]
7. [p ɔ r ʧ ʍ ɪ ŋ]
8. [l u ʃ: ɛ l f]
9. [g l æ ʃ : ɑ p]
10. [b æ ʃ: ɑ p]

C. Assimilation Nasality

1. [b ə n æ̃ n ə̃]
2. [m ʌ̃ ŋ k]
3. [m ɛ̃ n ʃ ə n]
4. [f r eɪ m ɪ̃ ŋ]
5. [n ʌ̃ m b ɚ]
6. [m ɪ̃ n ɪ̃ ŋ]

7. [m ɪ̃ n t aɪ m]
8. [h æ m ɚ̃]
9. [h ʌ n ɪ̃]
10. [m ɑ̃ m ɪ̃]
11. [n õʊ n]
12. [m ʌ̃ ŋ k i]

D. Combined Exercise

1. [n ɑ̃ɪ n̪ θ ɪ ŋ z]
2. [f ɔ r θ m ɔ̃ r n ɪ̃ ŋ]
3. [g l æ ʃ: ɛ l f]

4. [g l æ ʃ: t ɪ p]
5. [m ɛ̃ n ʃ ə n̪ ð ɛ m]
6. [l u ʃ ʧ eɪ n ʤ]

7. [m ɔ̃ r n d̥ ð ɛ m]   11. [m ĩ n ĩm aʊ s]
8. [w ɪ θ n̩ æ̃ n]   12. [h æ ʒ ʃ u z]
9. [p æ ʃ tʃ aɪ n i z]   13. [i t̪ ð ɛ r]
10. [m ɔ̃ r n ĩ ŋ æ n̩ t̪ θ ə m]   14. [m ẽɪ n̩ θ i m]

CHAPTER 14: CHANGES IN VOICING (pp. 52–53)

A. NARROW TRANSCRIPTION: VOICING CHANGES

1. [p l̥ eɪ t]   11. [k j u k ʌ m b ɚ]
2. [θ r̥ i]   12. [k l̥ ʌ s t ɚ]
3. [s t eɪ ʤ h̥ æ n d]   13. [l ɪ t̪ ɚ]
4. [p r̥ ɛ ʃ ɚ]   14. [k r̥ æ k ɚ]
5. [b ɪ t̪ ɚ]   15. [r oʊ h̥ aʊ s]
6. [b i h̥ aɪ n d]   16. [p l̥ i z]
7. [s l̥ i p i]   17. [k j u b ə]
8. [k l̥ ʌ b]   18. [eɪ t r̥ i j ə m]
9. [f r̥ eɪ d]   19. [m oʊ t̪ ɚ]
10. [r i h̥ ɚ s]   20. [f j̥ u d]

CHAPTER 15: ELISION/OMISSION AND ADDITION/EPENTHESIS (pp. 54–56)

A. SYLLABLE OMISSION

1. [v ɛ t ɚ ə n]   [v ɛ t r ə n]
2. [n æ ʃ ə n ʊ l]   [n æ ʃ n ə l]
3. [ɪ n t ɚ ɛs t]   [ɪ n t r ə s t]
4. [tʃ a k ə l ɛ t]   [tʃ a k l ə t]
5. [v ɛ ʤ ɪ t ə b ʊ l]   [v ɛ ʤ t ə b l̩]
6. [f ɛ d ɚ ʊ l]   [f ɛ d r ə l]
7. [r i z ə n ə b ʊ l]   [r i z n ə b l̩]
8. [f eɪ v ɔ r ɪ t]   [f eɪ v r ə t]
9. [s ɛ p ɚ ə t]   [s ɛ p r ə t]
10. [t ɛ m p ɚ ə tʃ ɚ]   [t ɛ m p r ə tʃ ɚ]

B. EPENTHESIS

1. [b i j i v l̩]   [b i ʔ i v l̩]
2. [g oʊ w aʊ t]   [g oʊ ʔ aʊ t]
3. [s i j ɪ t]   [s i ʔ ɪ t]
4. [s t eɪ j ɪ n]   [s t eɪ ʔ ɪ n]
5. [h aʊ w a r]   [h aʊ ʔ a r]
6. [s u w ʌ s]   [s u ʔ ʌ s]
7. [n u w eɪ l]   [n u ʔ eɪ l]
8. [t aɪ j ʌ p]   [t aɪ ʔ ʌ p]
9. [t u w æ p l̩ z]   [t u ʔ æ p l̩ z]
10. [j u w ɔ l]   [j u ʔ ɔ l]
11. [w i j i tʃ]   [w i ʔ i tʃ]
12. [t u w i z i]   [t u ʔ i z i]
13. [h i j ɔ l w eɪ z]   [h i ʔ ɔ l w eɪ z]
14. [h u w ɛ l s]   [h u ʔ ɛ l s]
15. [m eɪ j ɔ l s oʊ]   [m eɪ ʔ ɔ l s oʊ]

C. NASALS + INTRUSIVE STOPS

1. [w ɔ r m p θ]   6. [p r ɪ n t s]
2. [w ʌ n t s]   7. [æ n t s ɚ]
3. [h æ m p s t ɚ]   8. [ɛ m p f ə s ə s]
4. [t ɛ n t θ]   9. [k æ n t s l̩]
5. [s t r ɛ ŋ k θ]   10. [l ɛ ŋ k θ]

CHAPTER 16: ACCENT (pp. 59–61)

A. DISCRIMINATION

1. 2 Syllables: accent   boa   tearing   very   loaded   diphthongs   kitten
2. 1 Syllable: based   snows   kicked   dried   drowned   borne   branched
3. 5 Syllables: reactionary   disability   pronunciation   laryngology   unreality
4. 4 Syllables: dictionary   primarily   unaccented   approximate   exhalation
5. 3 Syllables: construction   syllable   nucleus   primary

B. WORD TRANSCRIPTION

1. [ə b 'z ɝ v d]
2. ['k æ t l̩]
3. ['ɔ r n ə ˌm ɛ n t]
4. ['f r ɪ k ʃ ə n]
5. [ʤ aɪ 'g æ n t ɪ k]
6. ['t ɛ l ə ˌf o n]
7. ['r aɪ d ɪ ŋ]
8. [k ə m 'p j u t ɚ]
9. ['f ɛ l oʊ]
10. [ˌs aɪ 'k ɑ l ə ʤ i]
11. ['ʤ ɛ n t l i]
12. ['d ɪ ʤ ə t l̩]
13. [ˌn e 'z æ l ə t i]
14. ['m ʌ f l ɚ]
15. ['l ɪ b ɚ ə l]
16. [ˌr ɪ 'm aɪ n d ə d]
17. ['ɪ n d ə ˌk e t]
18. [ə 'p ɪ r d]
19. ['k ɛ r ə k t ɚ]
20. ['p aʊ n d ɪ ŋ]
21. ['l æ ŋ g w ɪ ʤ]
22. ['s t æ n d ɚ d]
23. ['z aɪ l ə ˌf o n]
24. ['ʤ ɔɪ f ə l i]
25. [ˌɛ k s k l ə 'm eɪ ʃ ə n]
26. ['t ɛ l ə ˌv ɪ ʒ ə n]
27. ['m ɪ s t ɚ i]
28. ['h æ m b ɚ g ɚ]
29. [f ə 'n ɛ ˌt ɪ k s]
30. [k ə n 's ɝ v ə ˌt ɪ v]

CHAPTER 17: EMPHASIS AND INTONATION (pp. 62–64)

B. DISCRIMINATION

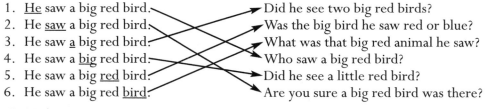

1. <u>He</u> saw a big red bird.   Did he see two big red birds?
2. He <u>saw</u> a big red bird.   Was the big bird he saw red or blue?
3. He saw <u>a</u> big red bird.   What was that big red animal he saw?
4. He saw a <u>big</u> red bird.   Who saw a big red bird?
5. He saw a big <u>red</u> bird.   Did he see a little red bird?
6. He saw a big red <u>bird</u>.   Are you sure a big red bird was there?

C. TRANSCRIPTION

1. We <u>did</u> it, but we didn't <u>want</u> to.
2. <u>They</u> arrived, and then <u>we</u> arrived.
3. We <u>drove</u> home, but they <u>walked</u> home.
4. They went on a <u>bus</u>, and we went on a <u>train</u>.
5. A <u>thesaurus</u> is like a <u>dictionary</u>.
6. A penny <u>saved</u> is a penny <u>earned</u>.
7. We came <u>early</u>, and they came <u>late</u>.
8. I <u>came</u>, I <u>saw</u>, I <u>conquered</u>.
9. The <u>spirit</u> is <u>willing</u>, but the <u>flesh</u> is <u>weak</u>.
10. He said <u>yes</u>, but he meant <u>no</u>.

D. MARKING INTONATION CONTOURS

1. Is this really the place?
2. They brought pretzels, hot dogs, potato chips, and beer.
3. Good morning! Is it time to go?
4. How many cookies do you want?
5. We're coming! We're coming! Wait a minute.
6. Mmmmmm, that's good.
7. Section thirteen is about computers.
8. Here today, gone tomorrow.
9. He said he was going where?
10. I guess that's the end of the chapter.

CHAPTER 18: TRANSCRIPTION OF CONNECTED SPEECH (pp. 65–66)

PHRASE AND SENTENCE RECOGNITION

1. Where's he going?
2. I'd like a burger and fries.
3. I saw some milk in the fridge.
4. When will he come?
5. We ate meat and potatoes for dinner.
6. It happened on the Fourth of July.
7. Is that a new hat?
8. I want you to come inside.
9. Who's he kidding?
10. How am I doing?
11. When's he leaving?
12. Did you want fries with that?
13. Busy as a bee.
14. Was he coming by train or bus?
15. I want a pizza with everything.

CHAPTER 19: DIALECTS AND /ɹ/ /ɝ/ /ɜ/ /ɚ/ (pp. 69–71)

C. WORD TRANSCRIPTION FROM SPELLING/DICTATION

1.	sermon	[s ɜ m ə n / sɝm ə n]	6.	after	[æftə/ æftɚ]
2.	avert	[ə v ɜ t /ə v ɝ t]	7.	learner	[l ɜ n ə/ lɝnɚ]
3.	desert	[d ɛ z ə t / d ɛ z ɚ t]	8.	shirker	[ʃ ɜ k ə/ʃ ɝ k ɚ]
4.	dessert	[d ə z ɜ t / d ə z ɝ t]	9.	water	[w ɑ t ə/ w ɑ t ɚ]
5.	furnace	[f ɜ n ə s / f ɝ n ə s]	10.	eastern	[i s t ə n / i s t ɚ n]

		[ɜ:]	[ɜ͡ə]
11.	cursed	[k ɜ : s t]	[k ɜ͡əs t]
12.	pearl	[p ɜ : l]	[p ɜ͡ə l]
13.	reserve	[r ɪ z ɜ : v]	[r ɪ z ɜ͡ə v]
14.	perch	[p ɜ : ʧ]	[p ɜ͡ə ʧ]
15.	servant	[s ɜ :v ə n t]	[s ɜ͡ə v ə n t]
16.	curbs	[k ɜ : b z]	[k ɜ͡ə b z]
17.	German	[ʤ ɜ : m ə n]	[ʤ ɜ͡ə m ə n]
18.	absurd	[æ b s ɜ : d]	[æ b s ɜ͡ə d]

		[ ]	[:]	[ə]
19.	farm	[f ɑ m]	[f ɑ : m]	[f ɑ ə m]
20.	corn	[k ɔ n]	[k ɔ : n]	[k ɔ ə n]
21.	pairs	[p ɛ z]	[p ɛ : z]	[p ɛ ə z]
22.	sure	[ʃ ʊ]	[ʃ ʊ:]	[ʃ ʊə]
23.	there	[ð ɛ]	[ð ɛ :]	[ð ɛ ə]
24.	are	[ɑ]	[ɑ :]	[ɑ ə]

/ə/ for postvocalic /r/

25.	hour	[aʊ ə]
26.	fire	[f aɪ ə]
27.	choir	[k w aɪ ə]
28.	sour	[s aʊ ə]
29.	spire	[s p aɪ ə]
30.	tower	[t aʊ ə][1]

---

[1]Intrusive /w/ may occur (e.g., [t a ʊ w ʊ l]).